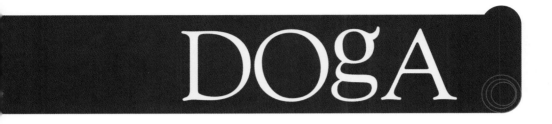

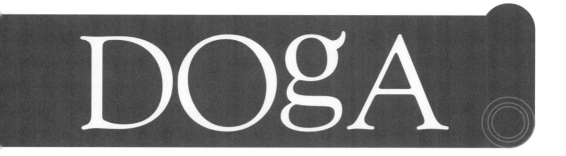

DOGA

Yoga for you and your dog

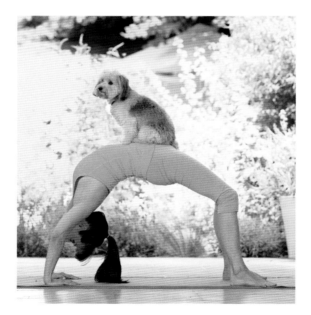

Mahny Djahanguiri

hamlyn

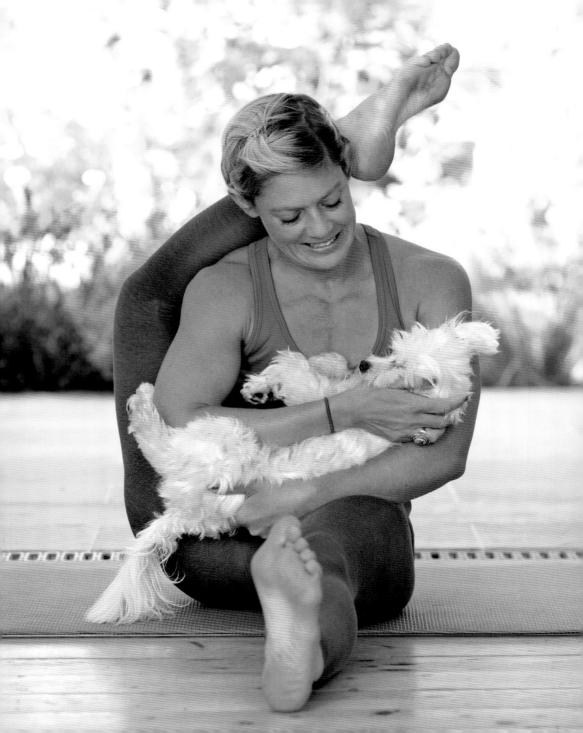

Contents

Introduction

Yoga is often described as the union of mind and body. Your body is your vehicle and, as with any vehicle, you need to maintain it well to keep it functioning in the best possible way. Many yoga teachers describe the mind as a chattering monkey, and the body can tighten up with stress when the mind isn't calm. In yoga, we focus on breath, movement and postures to help us shift our attention away from the mind, so that we can relieve tightness in our bodies. This helps to restore health and equilibrium to the whole body. The regular repetition of movements and postures helps to massage the joints so your body becomes flexible, light and strong. As you continue to practice yoga, the mind becomes more focused and steady.

Putting the Dog in Yoga

Robbie, my Maltese Terrier, is my best friend. He would follow me to the end of the world. When I come home from work, he'll be there to de-stress me, jumping up on my bed and showering me with kisses and licking my poor tired feet. He lavishes me with attention and affection and draws out some of my negative feelings which can, at times, be stressful for him too.

Before I discovered Doga, whenever I sat down on my mat to practise my yoga breathing, Robbie would immediately jolt up from the bed and climb on to my lap, playfully licking my face. I noticed a change in his attitude as be became more curious about the sound of my breath and the changes in my breathing pattern. I began incoporating him into my yoga practice and noticed how easily he bonded with me. I wanted to explore this interconnectedness and came up with various creative yoga postures and sequences in which you can involve your dog and that you will both benefit from.

Doga, Yoga and You

Doing yoga with your dog – and what better to call this than Doga? – can be highly challenging but exceptionally rewarding and fun. Of

*Doing yoga with
your dog is fun
and rewarding –
for both of you*

course dogs don't actually do yoga (although they can perform an awesome Downward Facing Dog when stretching in the morning), but they can get involved in the poses. Dogs get their exercise through other means, so unlike us they don't need the physical practice of yoga to achieve enlightenment. Our canine colleagues can reach nirvana during a walk in the park chasing squirrels. However, they do feed off our energy.

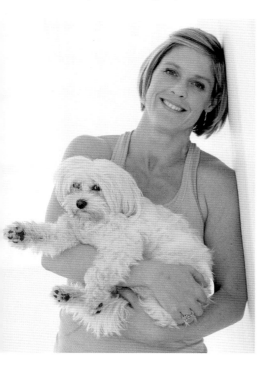

As a dog owner you'll know that when you're anxious, your dog seems agitated too. Similarly, when you are calm your dog relaxes, which is highly beneficial to his health and behaviour.

Sometimes I find too many people get too serious about yoga and forget it can be fun. Doga has very little to do with perfection. It brings laughter and joy to people's hearts as you tumble to the floor trying to maintain your balance, or are licked in the face while trying hard to relax in Corpse Pose. In Doga any-thing goes. There is space for freedom, fun and, most of all, bonding with your dog. To bond with your dog is to bond with nature and bonding with nature is yoga.

Your dog is the Dogi – a yoga participant or, sometimes, a yoga observer. You are the Yogi – a yoga practitioner. Together you create Doga – the union between dog and owner. Doga is a natural, symbiotic bonding exercise using the ancient tradition of yoga.

Chapter 1
The Yogi and the Dogi

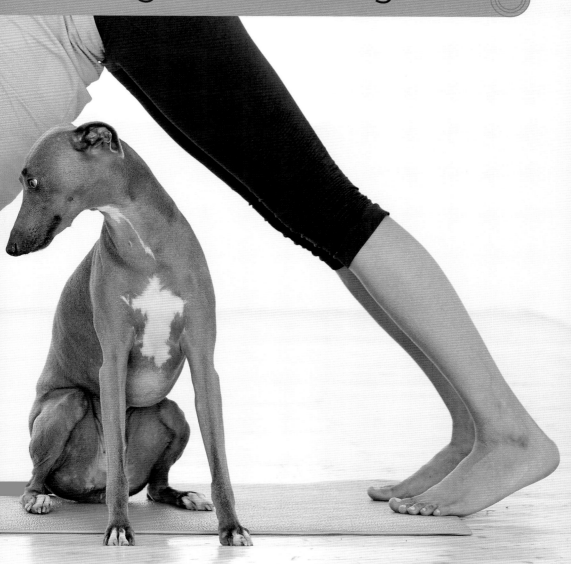

The Philosophy of Yoga

Ashtanga means 'eight limbs' in Sanskrit, which refers to the eight limbs of yoga as laid out in the Yoga Sutras – the teachings compiled by the sage Patanjali before the fifth century CE. These Sutras describe the philosophy, goals and techniques of yoga, and provide a road map to understanding the mind and how to liberate it. This road map includes The Eight Limbs of Yoga. This aphorism from the Sutras describes yoga perfectly: 'Yoga chitta vritti nirodha' ('Yoga is the cessation or control of the thought waves in the mind'). Unfortunately, controlling your mind can be a lot harder than it sounds. Much harder even than training a four-month-old puppy.

The Eight Limbs of Yoga

Much modern yoga focuses only on the third and fourth limbs of Patanjali's Sutras, which teach poses and breath control. However, six more limbs make up the foundation of yoga, and it's important that you understand them.

1 Yama

These five 'Moral Commandments' provide guidelines for how to behave towards others:
Ahimsa - Non-Violence
Satya - Truthfulness
Asteya - Non-stealing
Brahmacharya - Continence or Abstinence
Aparigraha - Non-coveting

2 Niyama

These five 'Observances' offer advice on how to behave ethically towards oneself.
Saucha - Purity
Santosha - Contentment
Tapas - Austerity
Svdhyaya - Study of the Self
Ishvara Pranidhana - Dedication to the Lord

3 Asana

The asanas are the yoga postures. Performing asanas purifies the internal and sense organs, oils the joints, stretches the muscles and realigns the skeletal body.

4 Pranayama

These breathing exercises make full use of the diaphragm, expand awareness, quieten the mind and keep the body strong.

5 Pratyahara

This refers to withdrawal of the senses. The first four limbs help you to bring physical and mental distractions under control, making it easier to draw the senses inwards to observe the Self.

6 Dharana

Dharana means concentration. With sense withdrawal, concentration follows. Your mind is now ready to focus on one point.

7 Dyana

The seventh limb is meditation, a state of absorption that arises from sustained concentration, free from intrusive thoughts. It cannot be forced. The aim of performing yoga poses is to ease the mind and strengthen the body in preparation for meditation.

8 Samadhi

Samadhi is the liberation from sufferings of the mind and body, achieved through transcending the meditative state of absorption. My teacher said it was like swimming in the ocean of pure love.

In Doga, our dogs become part of our meditation process, where we naturally apply the ethical codes of conduct that lead us to greater awareness of the oneness and harmony of nature.

Vinyasa

Using the correct breathing technique enables you to maintain a rhythm to your asana practice and build stamina and strength while clearing out toxins. The sequences of poses in this book have been carefully strung together to enable you to use your diaphragm to the fullest capacity.

Imagine each sequence as a pearl necklace. The string is the breath and the pearls are the postures. We use the thread of the breath to string on beads of postures, creating a necklace. This is called vinyasa, which means Movement/Breath synchronization. One vinyasa equals one inhalation or exhalation synchronized with one movement. The length of each breath dictates the length of each movement.

By following the correct vinyasa sequence, step by step, in the Standing and Seated Poses (See pages 34–71 and 72–95), you will steadily build up internal heat and strength. As you become more flexible and confident, you will be able to try more challenging poses.

Traditionally all yoga sequences end with inverted and restorative poses (See pages 124–31). Ending the yoga session with inverted poses helps restore and replenish the central nervous system, enabling the practitioner to prepare for meditation.

The Philosophy of Doga

When I'm walking my dog in the park, I sometimes invite fellow dog owners to a complimentary Doga class. They usually shake their heads, smile and give me one or both of the following replies:

Answer No. 1: My dog is far too nervous; he'll never sit still.
Answer No. 2: I can't touch my knees, let alone my toes.

I've got good news for you. You don't have to be flexible, and your dog doesn't have to be still.

What really matters is any yoga practice, whether it involves a dog or not, is following the ethical rules or moral commandments of classical yoga, as set out in the Yamas, the first limb of the sage Patanjali's Yoga Sutras (See page 10). These rules include:

Non-violence
❍ Never force your dog to do something he doesn't want to.
❍ During your yoga practice, avoid picking up your dog when he's asleep or when he's close to falling asleep – you wouldn't do that with a child either.
❍ Avoid picking him up when he's restless or wants to wriggle out of your grip.
❍ Your dog's tendons and ligaments, especially around the joints, are extremely sensitive and tender. If your dog weighs more than 5kg (11lb), avoid lifting him under his armpits: always support him with one hand under his tailbone and the other around his upper ribcage.
❍ Never over-stretch your dog – or yourself.

Truthfulness
❍ Avoid using treats to coax your dog into Doga. This is yoga, not a training session.
❍ If a yoga pose is too strenuous and your breath becomes uneven, be truthful with yourself and stop.

Non-stealing
❍ Avoid taking away your dog's personal space. If he wanders off to the other end of the room during your yoga practice, curls up in a ball and falls asleep, leave him be – that's perfectly OK. The goal of Doga is for your dog to absorb your calm, not to become stressed by the experience.

Contentment
❍ Be happy with what you have achieved today. It doesn't matter how far you got or which poses you have mastered: the fact that you took time out of your busy schedule to make space for yourself and your best friend is already an achievement in itself, so well done.

> *Doga is a symbiotic bonding exercise using the ancient tradition of yoga*

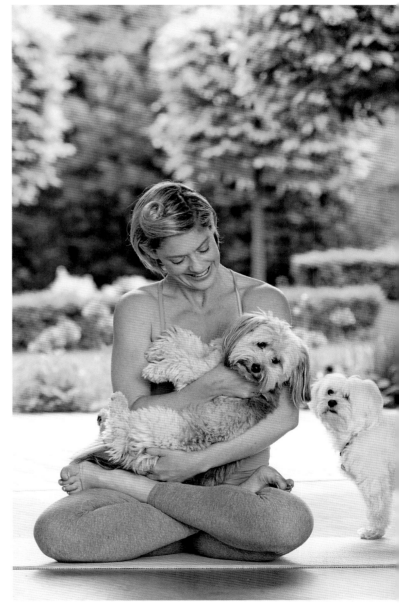

A few practical points before you start

○ Your practice should take place in a quiet environment, so try to make sure you will be undisturbed for at least 45 minutes. Switch off your phone and, if you can, your doorbell. Remember your dog's nervous system will calm down during your practice, and you don't want the sound of a buzzer to startle him.

○ Practise on an empty stomach. Wait at least two hours after a meal prior to your practice.

○ Before commencing Doga, seek advice from your vet if you have any concerns about your dog's health.

○ If you suffer from any health conditions yourself or have any injuries, consult your GP before starting yoga.

The Benefits of Doga

Although many people like to think of Doga as 'doggie yoga', this is not the case. In Doga, the Yogi does most of the hard yoga work while the Dogi is the by-stander and a sometime casual participant who aids you through the poses, serving as a weight or as yoga block or prop. In fact, because of your dog's anatomy and physiology, it would actually be harmful to stretch him out, as his tendons and ligaments are very tender.

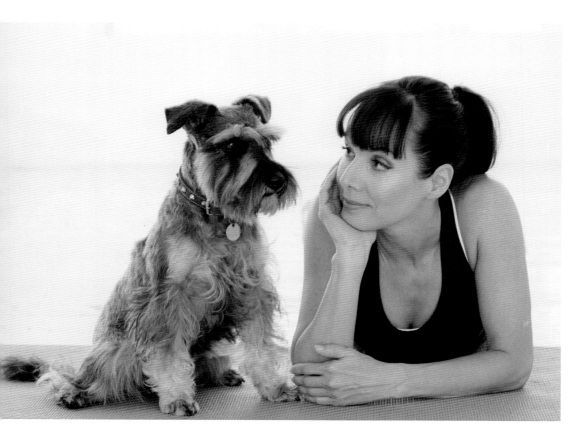

We don't want to rush things. Over time your dog will become used to you making space for yoga and encouraging him to join in. He will understand that this is a 'special time' where you can both relax and be together. Your dog doesn't even have to get involved in any of the yoga poses, but he can still absorb your calm. You can influence him through regulating your breathing pattern, which calms down your dog while also calming down your central nervous system.

Participating in Doga can have numerous benefits for your dog:

Deep sleep/absorbing calm

Dogs are thinking animals; they dream and can even have nightmares. Your dog's brain needs to process what he has seen and heard during the day, just like yours. A dog that lives in an especially stressful environment will find it hard to sleep. Without a good night's sleep, your dog can become moody, lethargic or even aggressive. After a Doga session, your dog will be out like a light, having absorbed your calm.

Trust

A regular yoga practice that involves positive affirmation, stroking and massage can enhance your dog's trust in you. If you are dealing with a traumatized dog, your peaceful and relaxed attitude will give him the reassurance he needs and not reinforce the negative attention he has received in the past.

A better bond between you

Doga enhances the natural bond that already exists between you and your dog. In Doga, we don't own our dog and our

weight – safety note

For your own safetey as well as that of your dog, the yoga postures and sequences in this book should only be practised if your dog weighs less than 5kg (11lb). As with any form of yoga practice, the first and most important guideline to follow is that of non-violence: do not harm yourself or others. Listen to your body and to your dog: if a pose feels wrong for either of you, stop.

dog doesn't own us. Instead we reconnect through intuition (as nature intended) rather than through intention. This helps your dog to bond with you naturally.

Reduced anxiety

For most dogs, the attachment they feel towards their owner is fundamental to their well-being. It is up to us to ensure that this attachment is not fear-based. Abandonment and attachment issues are increasingly common in dogs. By allowing your dog to come and go as he pleases on your yoga mat, Doga provides a great environment in which your dog can 'test' your boundaries, while you can reassure him that you are there for him.

Practising Doga also has many benefits for you, the Yogi, such as:

A better relationship with your dog

Stroking a pet releases hormones that help with anxiety and depression. Bonding with your dog on a regular basis allows you to unwind, providing room for creativity and curiosity to blossom. Your relationship with your dog is personal and sacred.

Doga helps you benefit from that unique relationship to an even greater degree.

Awareness

Through bonding with your dog, you will become more aware, seeing things as they are in their true form, without judgement. Observe how you conduct yourself next time you are in the park with your dog. Why not use awareness to help others clean up after their dogs, without being judgemental?

Mindfulness

Being mindful means living in the moment, with full awareness, without thinking of the past or the future. Like mother-and-baby yoga, Doga focuses our attention on something outside ourselves that we care about. We form a bond through intuition, using sound, massage and breathing techniques to become mindful of our dog. Mindfully stroking your dog may help you detect potentially harmful lumps and bumps that could have gone unnoticed.

Meditation

Meditation replenishes your central nervous system, helping you sleep and concentrate. It can alleviate anxiety and restores your body. Meditation is the union between the self and the beloved through

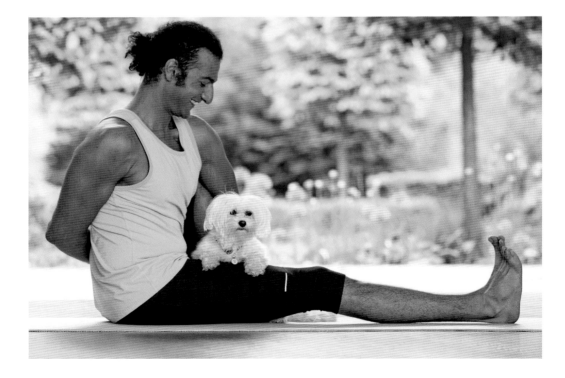

a state of Thoughtless Awareness, in which we are entirely in the present moment. In Doga, we don't have to meditate for hours to wait for this union to occur: our beloved is there. All we need to do is to turn our attention to our dog, with an open mind and an open heart. To shower your dog with unconditional love is being in a State of Bliss, which is what we hope to experience with meditation.

An extra weight and prop

Getting your dog involved in your yoga practice means having access to an extra weight or prop. His weight can challenge your strength and endurance, making your muscles work harder, and it can also help to deepen some of the more restorative and counterbalancing poses.

Your Approach

It is best to involve your dog gradually, rather than trying all the poses at once. A relaxed attitude will greatly improve your Doga practice: by ridding yourself of high expectations, you have the power to control whether or not this session will be enjoyable for you and your dog. A good exercise before you start your class is to ask yourself the following questions:

❍ What is my intention for today's Doga session? Do I want it to be fun and easy-going or tough and challenging?

❍ What do I need from this session to help me relax?

❍ How do I feel right now,?

❍ What would I like to transform within me?

Before each practice, focus on something you'd like to change. For example, if you are ambitious and have a stressful job, make small steps towards creating a more relaxed environment. Allow your dog to walk away or lick your face; embrace the moment by practising the art of letting go. It's a simple recipe, but letting go is really what Doga is all about.

Relaxing your mind

Below is a preparation exercise you can use if you find it hard to relax your mind:

Ignore your dog for a moment. Sit or lie down on your yoga mat and close your eyes. Ask yourself what you're feeling right now. Anger? Rage? Sadness? Can you locate the feeling in your body? Place your hand where the feeling is, inhale, then exhale sharply and let that feeling go. Repeat as many times as you need until that feeling has vanished. Remember, your dog will feel your transformation.

How to use this book

When you've completed the preparation exercise above, slowly move further into the physical part of the book, starting with Chapter 3 and moving forwards from there. You can try out individual poses at first until your dog feels comfortable and secure in the poses. When you both feel ready, you can try out some of the more challenging poses and sequences in Chapter 7. Remember to always finish with the restorative poses from Chapter 8. This will allow you to create a safe and calm platform for you and your dog to explore Doga in a creative, fun way.

Allow your dog to show you how Doga works. After all, our dogs are natural Yogis. They don't have an ego but can still put us to shame with their Downward Dog first thing in the morning.

LET'S DOGA!

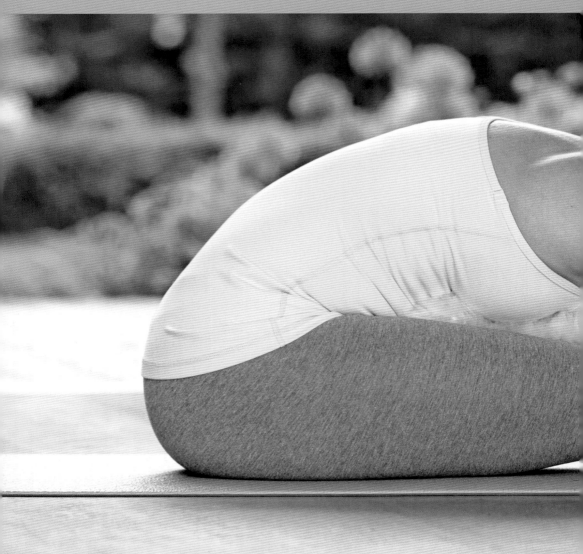

This chapter will help you prepare yourself and your dog for the practice of Doga poses and vinyasa sequences, through a series of excercises that will show you how to draw the senses inwards to ground and centre yourself through breathing and relaxation.

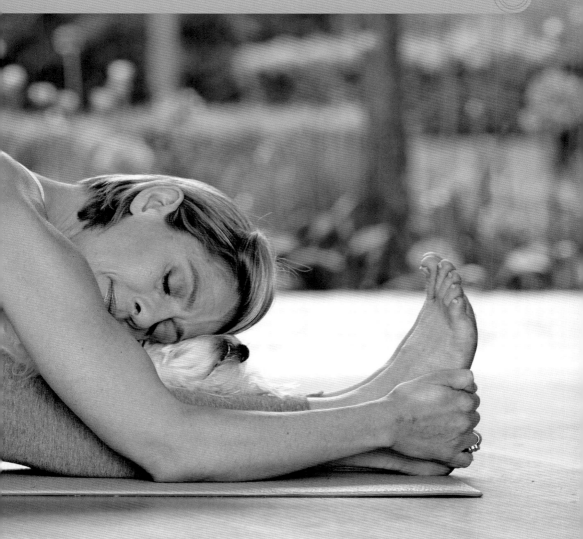

Starting Out

The First Steps

Relaxation ○ *Breath Awareness*

Like any kind of therapeutic mind–body work, one has to be fully grounded in order to reap the benefits of yoga.

Similar to mother-and-baby yoga, where the mother focuses on her own inner calm first before creating the 'bond' with her child, Doga focuses on the relationship between you and your dog.

Why is grounding oneself so important?

In this day and age people are not connected with nature as much as they once were. The stress and pace of modern day living, with its relentless barrage of information, can put a strain on our central nervous system, which governs sleep, digestion and overall mental, emotional and physical well-being. A good way to bring equilibrium into our daily lives is to ground ourselves with nature.

Helping you connect

As a dog owner I often ask myself these questions:

○ When was the last time I went out for a walk in the park with my dog Robbie without checking my messages on my mobile phone?

○ When was the last time I didn't run into the nearest coffee shop to get a quick 'caffeine fix' before walking my dog?

○ When was the last time I really relaxed with my dog, other than when sitting on the sofa watching television in the evening?

Does any of this sound familiar? Well, the first steps in Doga will help you to connect with your animal and rid yourself of day-to-day anxieties, making both of you feel better.

Getting grounded

In nature everything has roots, so let's start by lying down on the earth. Through 'gravity', earth – one of the four elements – can absorb any tension we hold in our bodies. In this posture, you can experience 'gravity' pulling you down into the earth.

Grounding is something you can do with your dog in the park, in your living room or in the garden. Find a secure place where you can't be disturbed and let your dog off the lead. Throughout the first two steps of grounding, try to ignore your dog as much as possible. Stay attentive to his or her behaviour, but try NOT to interact – keep focusing on you. This is your time.

There are three steps to grounding:

Step 1 Relaxation
Step 2 Breath awareness
Step 3 Connecting with your dog through your own breathing

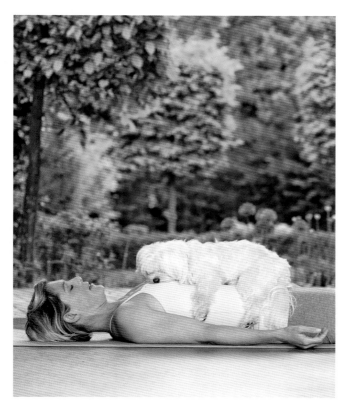

Step 1: Relaxation - (Savasana)

The Corpse Pose helps restore the central nervous system. Lie flat on your back, with your feet about 60cm (2ft) apart, palms facing upwards. Let your fingers and toes uncurl. Visualize a straight line from the crown of your head all the way through the centre axis of the spine down to your tail. Imagine you have a 'doggie tail'. On each exhale, lengthen your tail towards the front of the room. Relax your forehead, the root of your tongue, the back of your eyes and your inner ears.

Step 2: Breath Awareness

Now bring your awareness to your breathing. Allow the breath to travel in and out of your nostrils. Take long, deep breaths. Try to breathe from your abdomen, allowing your belly to rise on the inhalation and descend on the exhalation. If your dog comes to sit on your belly, enjoy his weight on your abdomen. After 10–12 minutes, slowly awaken your body and roll over onto your heart side, before slowly getting up into a seated position.

Step 3: Connecting with your Dog through your Breathing

Once you are in a seated position, move on to the breathing exercises on pages 22–5.

Mahny's observations

1   I've noticed in my classes that owners struggle with 'letting go of ownership' and this can be challenging, to say the least. The art of 'letting go' can also be extremely entertaining and funny. Don't be surprised if your dog starts furiously licking your face while you try hard to relax.

2   There's a mantra I like my clients to say to themselves three times: 'I am firmly grounded, earthed and centred into the bowels of this earth.'
    Say it over and over again until you feel it. Then gently observe what's going on outside of you. Is your dog restless or calm? What's going on for your dog? Again, remember not to judge. Be an observer.

The Panting Dog

The Fire Breath ○ *Kapalabhati Pranayama*

The third step in getting grounded is connecting with your dog through your breathing. While performing this exercise you're releasing unwanted toxins from your lungs as well as getting your dog's attention as you imitate his natural breathing pattern when panting. Your dog may become curious and think you're a dog, which is what you are after, as you want to coax your dog into your yoga practice.

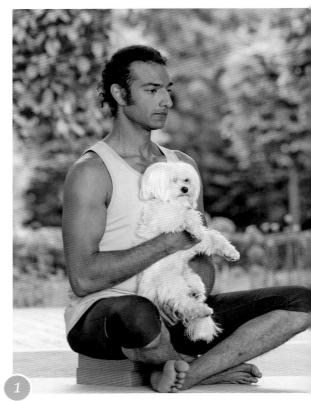

Using yoga blocks or a folded blanket for support, sit upright, crossed-legged, with a straight spine. Lift your dog up and slide one palm under his tailbone. With the other hand supporting his upper back, draw him close so that his spine is resting against your navel. Press your sitting bones firmly into the ground and lengthen your 'doggie tail'. ①

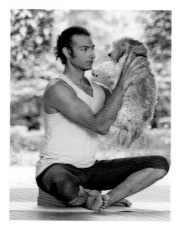

Modification

You can try turning your dog around so he faces you. Maintain eye contact with your dog while performing the same second step as below.

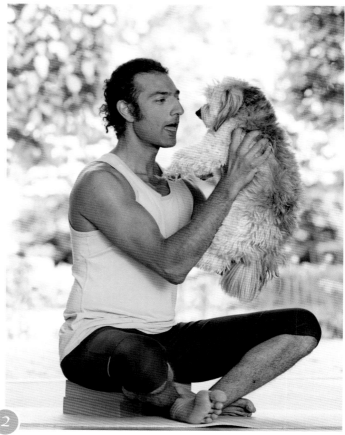

Now sharply exhale through your open mouth, slightly extending your tongue forwards (like a dog panting) as your abdomen draws towards the back of your spine. Inhale through an open mouth with your tongue out before repeating the sharp exhalation. This time, the exhalation should be much sharper, forceful and with sound. Focus on contracting your abdomen sharply as you exhale. Keep your spine still and long as you pant. If you start feeling nauseous, stop. Bend forwards and rest your head on the ground. Then repeat the cycle. Try to do this for a minute.

2

Ocean Breathing

Victorious Breath ○ *Ujjayi Pranayama*

Victorious breathing helps you lengthen your breath and regulates the exchange of oxygen with carbon dioxide in your blood. This has a calming effect on your nervous system and that of your dog. Try to use this type of breathing whenever you practise yoga, as it helps focus your attention on the present. Keeping the lips closed during the inhalation and exhalation requires practise: have a go for a minute; if you feel nausea or giddiness, stop and rest your head on a block.

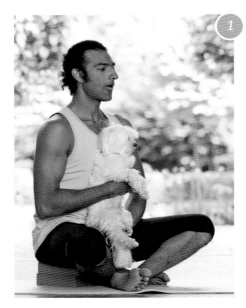

Sit upright in a crossed-legged position. As before, lift your dog up and slide one palm under his tailbone. With the other hand supporting his upper back, draw him close so that his spine is resting against your navel. This time, inhale through the nose, then exhale through a wide-open mouth. Direct the out-going breath slowly across the back of your mouth with a drawn out 'ha' sound. Repeat several times. Then close your mouth. As you inhale and exhale through your nose, direct your attention slowly towards the back of your throat, creating a soft 'rasping' sound.

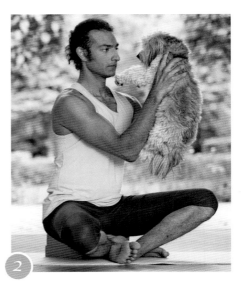

Turn your dog towards you, repeat Step 1 but keep eye contact with your dog. Your dog may become curious about your exhalation, as dogs are hypersensitive to sound and touch as well as the change in temperature and air pressure.

Lion Meets Dog

Lion Breath ○ *Shimasana*

The strong exhalation of the Lion Breath stimulates and awakens the spine. It is also an exercise to release emotional and mental stress, such as anger or sadness. The more you work your diaphragm, the more you exhale carbon dioxide, creating purer blood, which helps the kidneys, heart and lungs. We want our Doga practice to be lighthearted, vigorous and fun so it's vital to release as much tension as you can before you begin the poses and sequences.

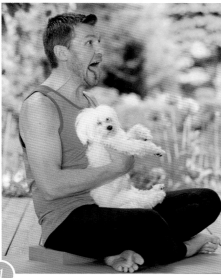

Sit upright in a crossed-legged position. Lift your dog up and slide one palm under his tailbone. With the other hand supporting his upper back, draw him close so that his spine is resting against your navel. Inhale sharply through both nostrils, then exhale and extend your tongue comfortably out of your mouth, curving it towards the chin. As you exhale, draw your abdomen wall in, widen your eyes, bare your teeth and stretch your facial muscles so that your face looks terrifying. Then release your abdomen and inhale smoothly through both nostrils, relaxing the facial muscles. Try 3–5 rounds; if you feel dizzy rest your head on a yoga block.

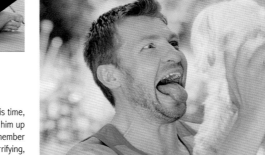

Again, sit in a crossed-legged position but, this time, slide your hands under your dog's armpit and lift him up so he is facing you. Keep firm eye contact and remember that, although you want to make your face terrifying, don't make it so scary that your dog wants to run away.

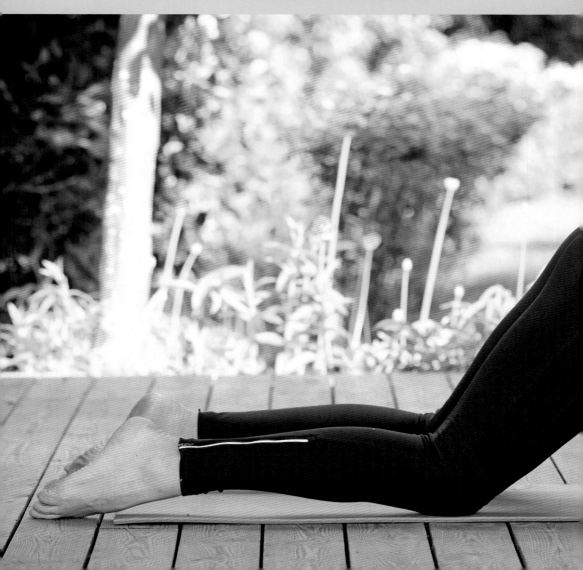

The Sun Salutation is a great physical warm-up, connecting breath with movement. This flowing sequence is traditionally practised in the morning, before breakfast. Together with your dog, you can wake up and warm up to the sun's rays and begin your Doga journey.

Chapter 3

Barking at the Sun

The Dawn of the Dog A

Sun Salutation Variation A ○ Suryanamaskar A

'Suryanamaskar' literally means 'to salute and worship the sun'. This is a flow-ing, fast-paced sequence and may be overwhelming at first, especially when lifting a dog, so I have given three modifications, which will ease your practice and help you build up strength. Sun Salutations not only require endurance, but patience. Your dog may wander off and that's fine – never force your dog to participate in Doga against his will (See page 12). This sequence gives you mental, physical and emotional stability. The more you do it, the easier it gets. Your dog will take to it in time. Try 3–5 rounds.

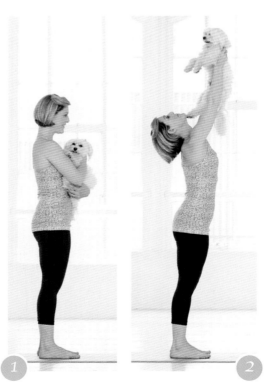

Mountain Pose (Tadasana)
Stand with your feet hip-distance apart. Root your feet, and imagine that you are extending your tailbone towards the ground and your crown is lifting upwards to the sky. Become still. Feel that you're standing evenly on both feet. Carry your dog close to your chest, sliding one hand under his tailbone and resting the other hand on the upper part of his back for support. Close your eyes and breathe deeply together with your dog.

Upward Salute (Urdhva Vrikshasana)
On an inhale, slide both hands under your dog's front legs and extend your arms over your head, looking up to your dog. Lift through the upper chest and draw your shoulder blades down and away from your ears; see if you can arch your mid-spine. This is a weight-bearing pose and requires strength, so you may want to keep your elbows slightly bent at the beginning.

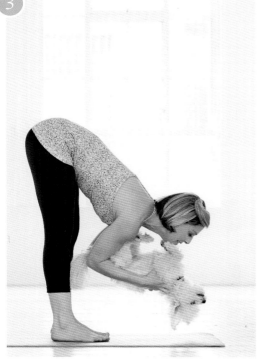

3

Standing Forward Bend (Uttanasana)

Exhale and fold deeply from your hip crease as you simultaneously fold your arms at the elbow joints, allowing your dog to rest on the inside of your forearms. Allow the weight of your dog to draw you down towards the ground. Bend your knees slightly if you feel discomfort in your lower back. Place your dog either flat on his front paws or on his back. Try to relax your neck in this position, as you massage your dog's neck.

4

Standing Half Forward Bend (Ardha Uttanasana)

Now place your dog on the front edge of your yoga mat. Press your palms or fingertips into the mat beside your dog. (You may have to shuffle your feet slightly forwards to get the right distance.) With an inhale, straighten your elbows and arch your torso away from your thighs. You might need to bend your knees slightly to help you get into this position. Look down your nose.

⑤ *Four-limbed Staff Pose (Chaturranga Dandasana)*

Keeping your shoulders stacked over your wrists, step back into plank position, with both legs and core engaged, and press firmly into your toes, keeping your upper and inner thighs engaged. Exhale, bend your arms, keeping your back straight and your upper arms pressed the into sides of your waistline as you lower down towards the floor.

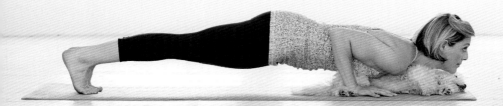

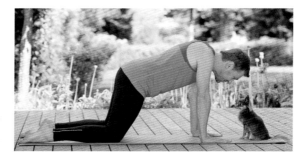

Modification

It is advisable to modify Four-limbed Staff Pose until you find the upper body and core strength to perform it fully. Ensure your shoulders are over the wrists and engage. Maintain this position as you drop both knees to the floor.

Now tuck your toes under and draw your shoulders blades together, pulling your elbows into your waistline as you drop your chest and then chin to the ground. Keep your sitting bones lifted. Make eye contact with your dog if he's still sitting in front of your mat.

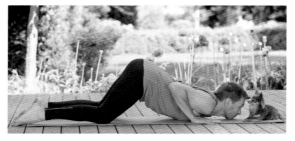

⑥ Upward Facing Dog
(Urdhva Mukha Svanasana)

Inhale, roll your toes over to touch the floor and, without letting the your thighs or knees touch the floor, come into Upward Facing Dog. Keep your legs engaged while pressing the tops of your feet down and dropping your hips. Make sure your shoulders stay stacked over your wrists, so you don't hunch.

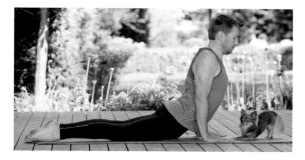

Modification 1

It can be difficult to keep your legs strongly suspended above the floor, so practise this modification first. From the knees-chest-chin position (See opposite page), release the tops of your feet to the floor and press them down. Slide your chest forwards and up, pressing the palms firmly into the floor until your arms straighten. Draw your shoulder blades together and engage your core. Keep your neck long and gaze down your nose.

Modification 2: Cobra

This posture is suited for those with weak lower backs or core stability problems. Keeping your navel on the ground, on an exhalation press through the palms of your hands and extend your toes back. Inhale, roll your shoulders back and lift your chest higher, like a serpent. Don't strain your neck. Keep your elbows bent.

7 Downward Facing Dog (Adho Mukha Svanasana)

With an exhalation, push your thighs back and straighten your legs, but be sure not to lock the knees. Press your fingertips into the floor. Draw your shoulder blades apart and down towards the waistline. As you lift your sitting bones up towards the ceiling, imagine you were a dog strung upside-down from his tail. Keep your head between your upper arms; don't let it hang. Stay there for 5 breaths.

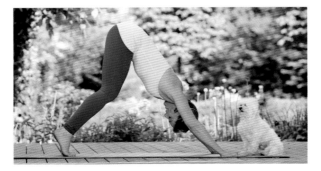

Modification: The Puppy Pose

This modification is suited to practitioners with tight hamstrings and tight lower backs. Instead of keeping your legs straight, keep the knees bent and your heels slightly lifted away from the floor. Keep your hands shoulder-distance apart, with wrists and index finger slightly turned out to avoid any strain in wrists and rotator cuffs. Relax your head and gaze at the floor.

8 On an exhale, bend your knees and look between your hands. Inhale, step your feet forward between your hands, returning to your position in Step 4. Exhale and fold forwards from your hip crease, releasing the palms of your hands on your dog. If you are super-flexible release your neck and rest your head on your dog. If you're tight in the hamstrings, bend your knees. With both hands, massage your dog for a few breaths, then lift your arms back up into Step 2 (Upward Salute).

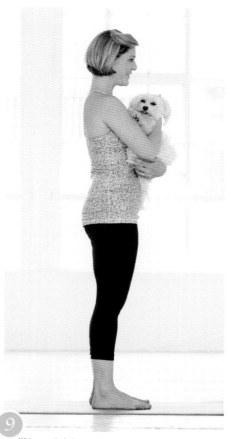

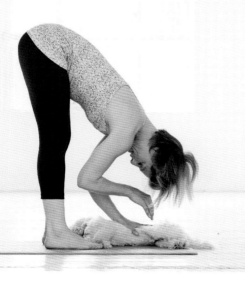

9 With an exhalation, return to Step 1 (Mountain Pose).

Flexing and extending the spine helps develop your core stability

Through standing poses, you build a core foundation from the feet upwards, gaining flexibility and strength. Your dog's weight will help you to maintain your equilibrium and poise. Together you stand the test of endurance through the more challenging standing vinyasa sequence.

Chapter 4

On Two Paws

The Loose Dog

Standing Forward Bend ○ *Uttanasana*

Standing Forward Bend will awaken your hamstrings and soothe the mind.
It's the ultimate bonding pose, as your dog will be held in a back bend, which
requires trust and patience. In this pose you counterbalance each other. As
your dog acts as a weight to deepen the stretch, your function is to reassure
him. Keep eye contact throughout the pose. Support your dog with both
your hands, one on his sacrum and the other under the nape of his neck.

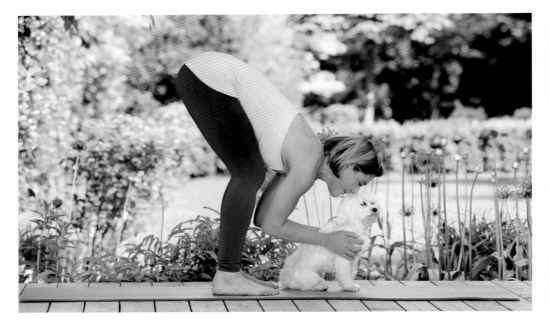

Modification

If you're a beginner or you suffer from lower-back issues, put your dog down
on the floor and bend your knees so your knees are stacked over your ankle
bone. This is a great opportunity to pet your dog. If he's lying on his back,
give him a belly rub or, if he prefers to lie on his belly, stroke him from top to
tail and/or give him a nice neck massage (See page 134).

Advanced

Exhale, bend from your hips, folding forwards. Maintain length through the front of your torso and keep the knees relaxed. When you reach your maximum stretch, let the weight of your dog do the work for you. Relax your neck and stay in the pose until your dog wriggles out of the pose or your legs begin to shake.

Your dog helps you relax into this pose

The Dog in a Chair

Chair Pose ○ *Utkatasana*

This posture requires strength and stamina; it's a great pose for expanding the breath. It is similar to sitting in a chair, except you have to balance yourself without a chair. Your dog acts as a weight to help you work your inner-thigh muscles and abdomen. At the same time your dog can sense your powerful and fierce breath, which affects his nervous system. In this pose your dog gets a full stretch through the lower spine and a release through the tight hind legs.

Beginners

If you're a beginner or suffer from lower-back issues, keep your feet hip-distance apart. Bend your knees and sit deep into an imaginary chair, lengthening your tailbone towards the ground. Ensure your knees are stacked firmly over the ankle bones without twisting. Keep your dog close to your chest and support him like a baby. Keep focusing on lengthening the exhalation, while extending your tailbone towards the floor.

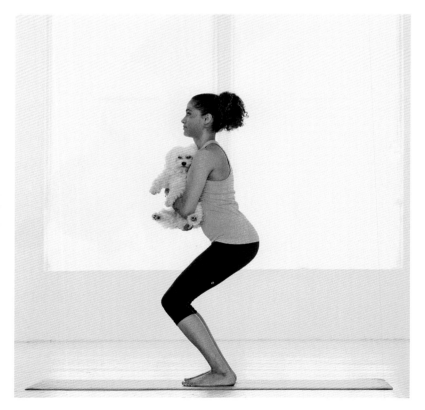

modification

The more you lower your tailbone to the ground in Chair Pose, the more challenging it becomes. To strengthen your thighs, try squeezing a yoga block between your knees while you perfom this pose.

safety note

If your dog is weighs more than 4kg (8lb 13oz) you must practise the beginner's version of this pose at all times to avoid any lower-back pain or neck strain.

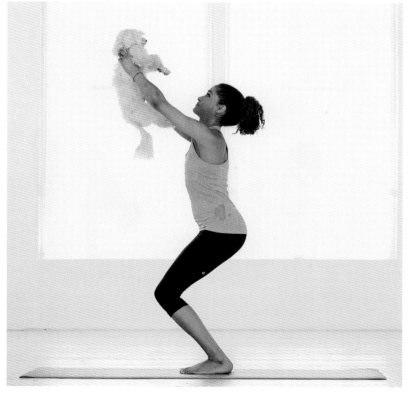

Advanced

Stand with your big toes touching and your heels slightly apart. Bend your knees and sit deep into an imaginary chair, lengthening your tailbone towards the ground and keeping your knees and ankles pressed together. Inhale and lift your dog up in the air, keeping both arms straight. Look up into your dog's face and breathe deeply from your abdomen. Hold for 3–5 breaths. Try not to strain your neck or face.

Up and Down the Mountain

Standing Forward Bend and Chair Pose sequence ○
Uttanasana and Utkatasana sequence

Designed to warm up and strengthen the spine, this invigorating sequence is a great way to start the day – especially when you know you'll be sitting at your desk for nine hours. Moving from Mountain Pose (See page 28) into Standing Forward Bend (See page 29) and then through to Chair Pose (See pages 38–9) activates the deep-seated lower-back muscles, quads and inner thighs, all of which support the spine, keeping it strong and vital.

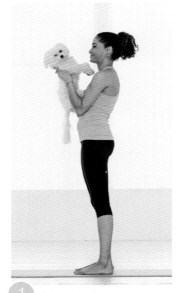

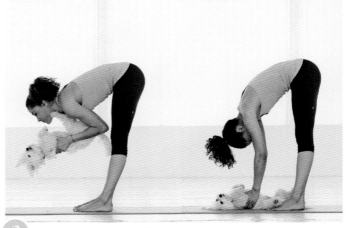

1 *Mountain Pose
(Tadasana)*
Stand in Mountain Pose with your dog facing you and your feet hip-distance apart. Hold your dog like a baby close to your chest.

2 *Standing Forward Bend (Uttanasana)*
Exhale and bend from your hips. Be sure not to lock your knees and come into Standing Forward Bend.

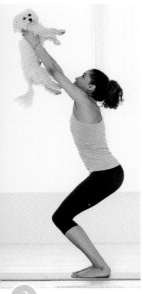

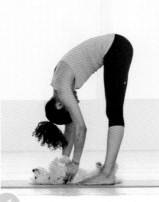

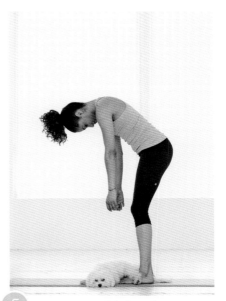

③ *Chair Pose*
(Utkanasana)
Exhale, bend your knees
and squat. Inhale and lift
your dog up over your
head into Chair Pose. Hold
for 3–5 breaths.

④ *Standing Forward Bend*
(Uttanasana)
Exhale, fold forwards and come into
Standing Forward Bend. Stay in this
pose for as long as is comfortable.

⑤ *Mountain Pose (Tadasana)*
Place your dog on the ground. Gently roll
up into Mountain Pose, keeping your knees
soft and stacked over the ankle bones.

Remain for a few breaths in Mountain
Pose, mentally rooting yourself through
the front balls and heels of your feet.
Repeat when you both are ready.

The Lunging Hound

Warrior Lunge ○ *Anjaneyasana*

Warrior Lunge, sometimes called Crescent Lunge, is a dynamic standing pose that strengthens and stretches the muscles in your entire body. It also stabilizes mind and body and purifies the internal organs by activating the internal *agni* (heat/fire) of the digestive system. Your dog acts as a weight, making the pose more demanding. If you're not strong and stable through this pose, your dog will be unstable too. Your firm and direct concentration on your dog will rub off on him, making him more submissive for later poses.

Advanced

With your left leg, come onto the ball of your foot so your back heel is arching. Imagine you are pressing your back heel into a wall. Now engage your core, breathing deeply. Holding your dog securely in your arms and maintaining a strong, stable core, on an inhalation, sweep your dog over your head, with strong extended arms, shoulder blades drawn away from your ears. Look up at your dog and maintain eye contact. If your dog wants to come down, bend your back leg and gently release him onto the floor.

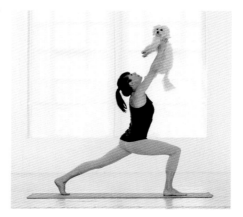

Modification

If you're a beginner or suffer from weak lower back and core strength, support yourself by bringing your back knee to the floor (you can slide a folded blanket underneath) and untucking your toes. Place your dog on your knee so that he is facing you. Support him under his forelegs. Keep your shoulders and hips aligned and don't twist your front knee. Breathe deeply, keeping your gaze steady and fixed on your dog so as not to lose balance.

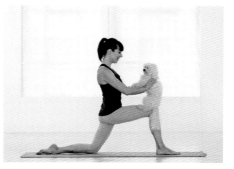

The Running Hound

Runner's Lunge ○ *Alanasana*

This Runner's Lunge acts as a counterpose to the previous poses.
It brings flexibility through the hips and groins, as internal heat gets released
through the groin muscles and calves. It also gives your dog an opportunity
to come down from the high Warrior Lunge and rest on his back, feeling your
deep exhalation as you counteract the pose.

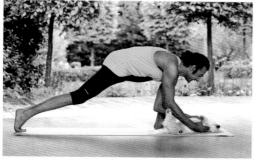

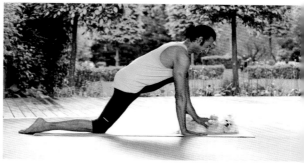

High

Bring your weight through the front torso as if lunging forwards
(like a runner preparing for a sprint). Take the weight onto your
back foot, with your toes tucked under. Transfer most of the
weight onto the toes, shifting your pelvis forwards and releasing
the tailbone towards the ground. Engage your core and take both
hands into the in-step of your inner left heel. Rest on both hands
(or you can bend further onto your forearm) with your dog between
your hands (your dog is either lying on his back or resting on his
front paws). If you have the flexibility, try to rest your head on your
dog. In this pose your dog aids as a yoga block. Breathe deeply for
as long as you can, and focus on the exhalation. Your dog should
absorb your peace. Take the opportunity to massage your dog.

Low

For the low version of the this lunge, bend your back leg and lower
your knee to the floor, then release both hands to the floor. Try to
soften your neck as you place one hand on your dog to give him
a massage.

observation

*I find my dog calms down instantly in this
posture because he can feel the force of my
breath when I succumb and release into this
deep therapeutic counterpose that is designed
to soothe my sympathetic nervous system, which
is responsible for my 'fight or flight' trigger.*

The Resting Dog

Child's Pose ○ *Balasana*

This pose helps you to relieve stress and fatigue, making it the ultimate restorative pose. It also helps to alleviate back and neck pain. You can come into Child's Pose every time you feel you want to have a rest between poses. Your dog can be your yoga block, making this the ultimate Doga 'bonding' pose. Depending on your flexibility, one great way to relax is to rest your forehead on your dog's navel. Feeling his breathing and heartbeat at the same time makes this a unique moment for Yogi and Dogi.

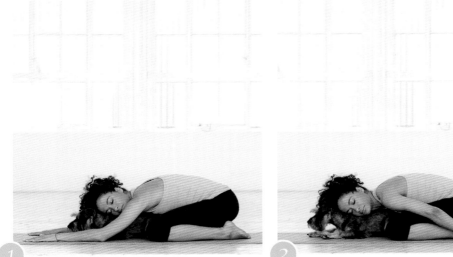

1 Bring your dog between your thighs to a position in which you are able to fall forwards over your dog. Engage your inner thigh muscle as you drive your sitting bones back towards your heels. Fall forwards from your hips. Gently connect your torso with the back of your dog, being careful not to rest your weight on him.

2 With a larger dog, you can rest your hands forward and rest your head on the nape of his neck, almost 'melting' over him. Having your arms forward gives you more release of your shoulders. With smaller dogs, you can have your arms back.

In this calming
pose, Yogi and
Dogi relax as one

If your dog is happy to
allow it, you can have him
as a weight on your lumbar.

3

The Dawn of the Dog B

Sun Salutation Variation B ○ *Suryanamaskar B*

This is a slightly more advanced variation of Dawn of the Dog A, the Sun Salutation sequence desribed on pages 28–33. It incorporates low and high lunges, which will open the hips and groins and help build core strength. Make sure you have mastered the first version before attempting this variation, which requires strength, stamina and breath control. However, you can always take a rest in Child's Pose (See pages 44–5) before repeating the sequence on the opposite side.

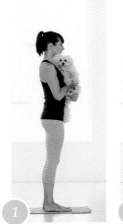

1

Mountain Pose (Tadasana)
Stand in Mountain Pose with your feet hip-distance apart.

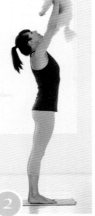

2

Upward Salute (Urdhva Vrikshanasa)
On an inhale, slide both hands under your dog's front legs, and extend both your arms over your head, looking up to your dog.

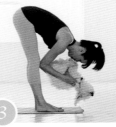

3

Standing Forward Bend (Uttanasa)
Exhale and fold deeply from your hip crease as you simultaneously fold your arms at your elbow joints, allowing your dog to rest on the inside of your forearms.

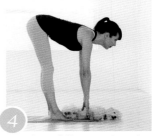

4

Standing Half Forward Bend (Ardha Uttanasa)
Rest your dog on the floor between your hands. Inhale and roll onto the tips of your fingers.

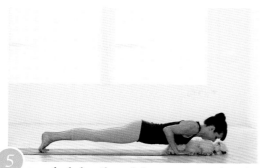

5 *Four-limbed Staff Pose (Chaturranga Dandasana)*
Exhale, step back into Four-limbed Staff Pose keeping the weight forwards as you bend your arms with a straight back or following the Modification (See page 30).

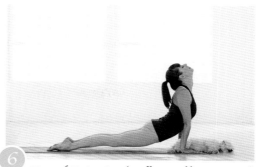

6 *Upward Facing Dog (Urdhva Mukha Svanasana)*
Inhale and roll over toes, without dropping the knees or the pelvis on the floor, into Upward Facing Dog.

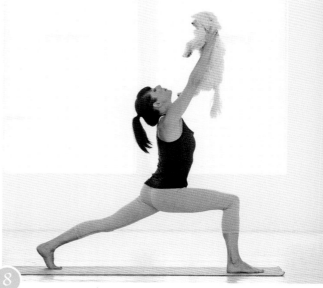

7 *Downward Facing Dog (Ardho Mukha Svanasana)*
Exhale, shift your weight back and lift the sitting bones towards the ceiling into Downward Facing Dog, keeping your weight evenly distributed through all four limbs.

8 *Warrior Lunge (Anjaneyasana)*
Exhale and step your right foot forwards between your hands. Pick your dog up off the floor. Inhale and sweep your dog over your head, looking straight up at him.

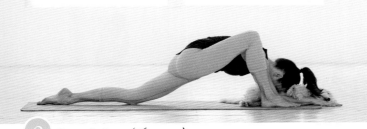

Runner's Lunge (Alanasana)

Exhale, bend your back knee and place your dog on the ground, close to the inside of your right heel. Lunge further forwards, resting your head on your dog if you can.

9

Child's Pose (Balasana)

10

Take your right leg back. Exhale and sit back, resting your sitting bones on your heels. Surrender into Child's Pose and stay there as long as is comfortable or until you are ready to repeat the sequence on the left side.

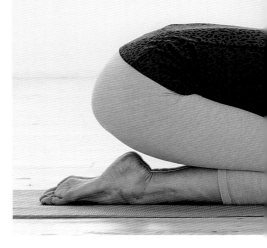

*Child's Pose is
always available to
us when we need it*

You and Me Makes Three

Extended Triangle Pose and Revolved Triangl Pose ○
Utthita Trikonasana and Parivrtta Trikonasana

Extended triangle pose stretches and strengthens the thighs, knees and ankles; it also stimulates the abdominal organs and helps alleviate stress. Your dog acts as a weight and also reminds you to keep your waistline long. He has the chance to feel your ribcage expanding and contracting; this movement of the ribcage and intercostal muscles stimulates and massages your dog's inner organs. Revolved Triangle pose stretches your legs, opens your hips and twists your torso. It acts as a counterpose to the Extended Triangle Pose. In this posture your dog is passively acting as a yoga block while receiving a gentle massage from you. If he wanders off, just continue with the sequence.

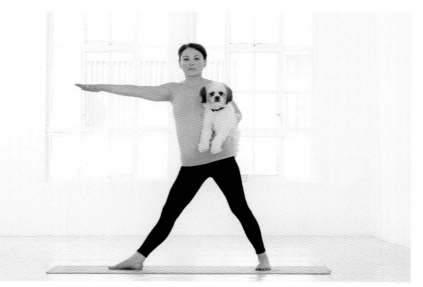

1 Standing sideways on your mat with your feet 1–1.2m (3½–4 feet) apart, raise your right arm so that it is parallel to the floor while your left hand supports your dog's upper body. Slide him on top of your left hip, making sure he is positioned comfortably. Turn your left foot in slightly and your right foot out to the right at 90 degrees from your thighs and turn your right thigh outwards, so that the centre of the right kneecap is in line with the centre of the right ankle.

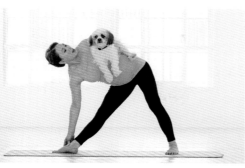

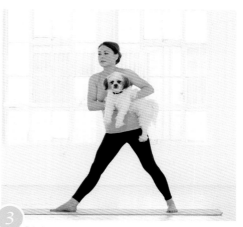

2 **Extended Triangle Pose (Utthita Trikonasana)**
Exhale and extend your torso out to the right and rotate your torso to the left. Rest your right hand on your foot or shin, wherever is comfortable – making sure to keep the two sides of your torso equally long. If you feel your dog is uncomfortable or not sitting correctly, slide him further up along your waistline until you think he's fully supported. Turn your head up, looking at your dog, making eye-to-eye contact. Don't strain your neck in this pose and hold for 5 breaths. Inhale and come back up, then repeat on the other side. If your dog wants to jump off, let him wander off for a while.

3 Exhale and come back up. Pivot the hips and torso to square them up with the front of the mat so that the heel of your back foot is in line with that of your front foot, with the toes of your front foot pointed forwards and your back foot at a 45-degree angle.

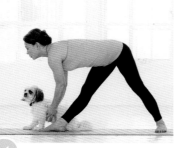

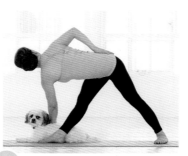

4 Extend your right arm out to the side at shoulder level and hold your dog with your left hand. Exhale and fold from your hips, but continue to extend through both sides of the waistline. Place your dog on the floor about 5cm (2in) away from the outer heel of your right foot.

5 **Revolved Triangle Pose (Parivrtta Trikonasana)**
Reach with your left hand to stroke your dog and place your right hand on your tailbone. Shift your weight onto your right foot. Inhale and look over your right shoulder, without straining your neck and eyes.

6 Finish with Wide-legged Forward Bend (see pages 54–5). Either rest your dog on the floor and give him a belly rub or, if you want to go further, bend your knees, resting your dog on his back and release the crown of your head on your dog's belly without pressing into it. This pose releases tight hamstrings, soothes the mind, with the head below the level of the heart, and calms your dog's nervous system.

The Brave Hound

Warrior 1 and 2 ○ *Virabhadrasana 1 and 2*

Virabhadra means 'fierce warrior'. It may seem odd to give a yoga pose such a name when we practise non-violence, but in yoga, 'fierce' means 'courageous'. What we are really performing here is the pose of the spiritual warrior who bravely does battle with the universal enemy, self-ignorance, and the ultimate source of all our sufferings. This pose stretches the chest and lungs, making this a 'courageous heart-opening' pose.

When you are performing the Warrior poses, the weight of your dog helps you to maintain strength through your upper back and legs but most importantly your dog aids as a reminder of how firm and rooted your legs and feet must be in order to maintain stability and not lose balance or concentration.

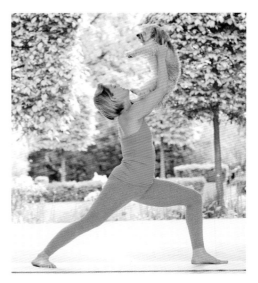

Warrior 1

Stand sideways on your mat with your feet parallel, approximately 1.5m (5ft) apart. Turn your right foot slightly to the left and turn your left foot out to the left at 90 degrees. Make sure the heels are in line with each other. Rotate your torso to the left, squaring the front of the pelvis as much as possible with the front edge of your mat. With your right heel firmly anchored to the floor, bend your left knee over the left ankle. With both hands supporting your dog's upper torso, sweep him over your head so you can look straight at him. Keep your chest lifted and your legs and arms strong. Stay for as long as you can, until your breath and legs feel shaky.

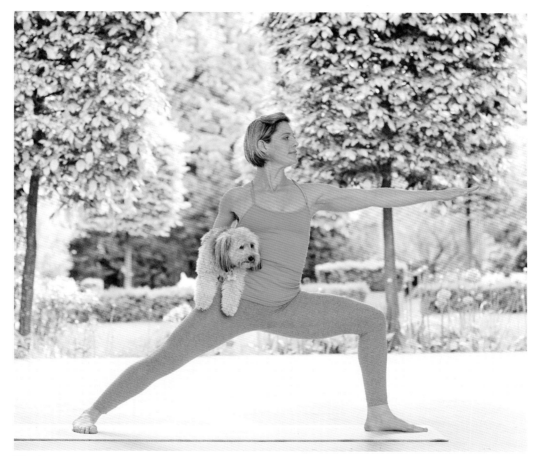

Warrior 2

Stand sideways on your mat with your feet parallel, approximately 1.5m (5ft) apart, and your dog resting on your upper right hip. Turn your right foot slightly to the left and turn your left foot out to the left at 90 degrees. Make sure the heels are in line with each other. Exhale and bend your left knee so it's stacked over your left ankle. Keep pressing the outer right heel firmly into the floor. Raise your left arm so that it is parallel to the floor and reach actively out to the left, shoulder blades wide, and palm down. See if you can gaze past your left third finger. Breathe deeply so your dog can feel your ribcage expanding and contracting.

Trust in Me

Wide-legged forward bend ○ *Prasaríta Padottanasana*

This pose strengthens your legs and opens the shoulders. It also challenges your ability to maintain stability through the balls of your feet and your heels, thereby opening up the backs of your legs and hamstrings. This position involves your dog lying on his back. Again, this is a matter of trust and can calm them down, but some longer-torsoed dogs, like dachshunds, may prefer to be on their front. You will find that having your dog in your arms gives your lower back muscles and legs more of a stretch than the poochless version of this pose.

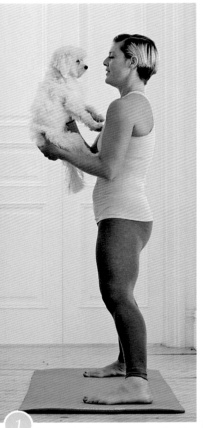

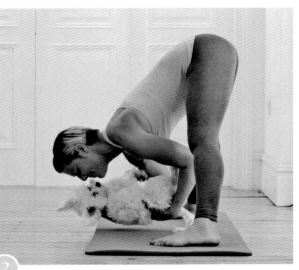

1 Take your dog in your arms, supporting his back and sternum. Bring him level with your face so he can sense your breathing. Step your feet out wide on the mat.

2 Exhale and bend from the hips, leaning forwards. Maintain the length of the front torso. Make sure you support your dog's back and maintain eye contact. Take a few breaths when you reach the lowest point you can.

*This pose stretches
the hamstrings
and calms
the mind*

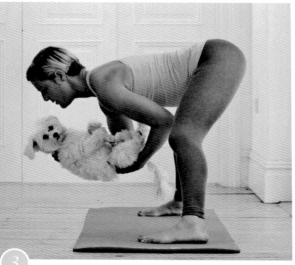

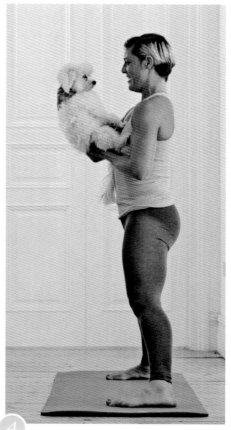

3 Stay in this position as for as long as both you and the dog feel comfortable, maintaining eye contact so he feels safe. If your dog starts wriggling, your breath becomes unsteady or you feel any kind of tightness, it's time to release the pose: bend your knees; press to the outer edges of your feet, engage your core; inhale and come up.

4 When you're back upright, exhale (smile at your dog!). Keep breathing and make sure your dog is relaxed and happy. It's a good idea to let him have five minutes to wander around on his own until he's ready to interact with you once more.

Brave Heart
Meets Brave Hound

Warrior sequence ○ *Virabhadrasana sequence*

This sequence builds you up from the ground upwards: you will stretch and strengthen your feet and ankles and tone your core muscles as well as your legs and your arms. The transition from Warrior 1 into Warror 2 expands the chest and helps you to deepen your breathing. Ending with a Forward Bend releases the hips, back and neck in preparation for more advanced backbends.

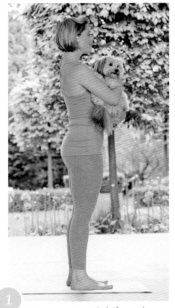

Mountain Pose (Tadasana)
Come into Mountain Pose, holding your dog like a baby close to your chest.

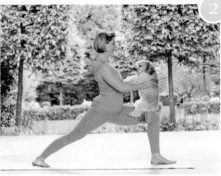

2 Exhale and step back your right leg about 1–1.2m (3½–4ft) back. Make sure your hips stay square and in line with the front of the mat as you settle your right heel on the ground. Bend your left knee. Place your dog on your left knee.

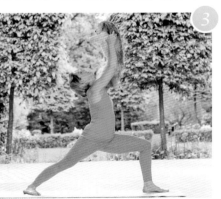

3 *Warrior 1 (Virabhadrasana 1)*
Inhale and sweep your dog up with extended arms. Stay in Warrior I as long as is comfortable. Exhale and release your dog onto your knee.

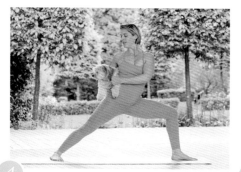

4   Now change the position of your dog, by pivoting your hips to the right side. Press into the outer right heel and simultaneously swing your dog over to the other side, placing him between your upper right hip and torso.

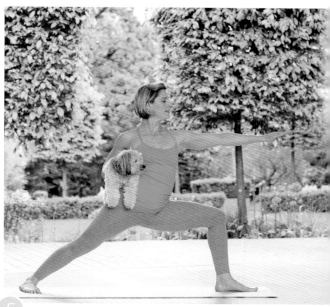

5   *Warrior 2 (Virabhadrasana 2)*
Exhale, press firmly into the outer right foot as you bend the left knee, engaging the inner arch of your left foot. Extend your left arm, palm facing downwards.

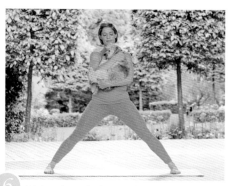

6   Inhale and come back up with feet parallel and your dog close to your chest. To complete the sequence, exhale and bend forward from your waist.

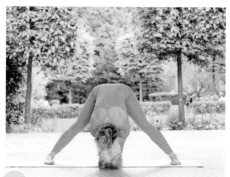

7   *Wide-legged Forward Bend*
(Prasarita Padottanasana)
Release your dog on to the mat and rest your hands on him. Stay in this pose for as long as you need to.

Growing Together

This is a balancing pose, which prepares you for meditation by allowing you to concentrate on one point. The balancing helps you to learn about your core – where the weaknesses are on each side. You'll find your dog really helps you as a counterbalance.

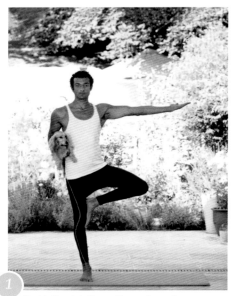

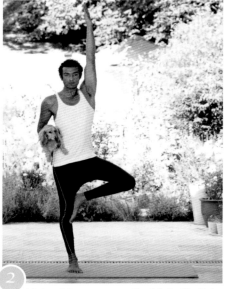

1 Start in Mountain Pose, with your dog resting on your right hip. Ensure that your arm is fully underneath your dog, supporting him – you should feel his weight on your forearm. You want to be perfectly straight, so you may wish to hold him higher than your hip. Bring the heel of your left foot up as high as it will go and place the sole of the foot on the inner right thigh, but don't press the heel into your kneecap – rest your foot either above or below your knee.

2 Inhale and draw your arm up. Your left shoulder blade should move downwards as you extend your arm. Maintain integrity and length in the spine. Repeat on the opposite side if your dog is still relaxed and happy.

Branching Out

Extended Hand to Big Toe Pose ○
Utthita-hasta-padangustasana

This is a more advanced variation of the classic Tree pose shown opposite, requiring flexibility in your hips and shoulders. With the help of your dog's weight on the opposite side to your raised leg, you'll find it easier to balance. Standing balancing poses such as this one strengthen the legs and ankles, stretch the hamstrings and promote balance and focus in both you and your dog.

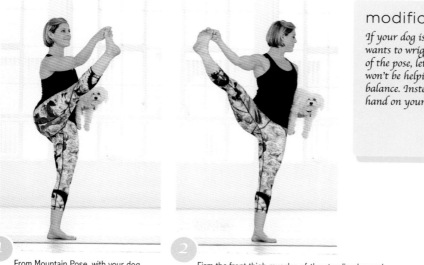

modification

If your dog is restless and wants to wriggle himself out of the pose, let him go, as he won't be helping you with the balance. Instead, keep one hand on your hip for support.

1 From Mountain Pose, with your dog resting on your left hip, reach your right arm inside your right thigh and grab hold of your big toe. Exhale, and extend your right leg forwards, straightening the knee as much as possible. Hold for 30 seconds.

2 Firm the front thigh muscles of the standing leg and press the outer thigh inwards, then on an exhale swing the raised leg out to the side (without lifting the right hip). Look over your left shoulder. Hold for 30 seconds, then swing the leg back to the centre on an inhale and release the leg down on an exhale. Repeat the whole sequence again on the left side.

The Hip Sitter

Extended side angle stretch ○ *Uthita Parsvakonasana*

This stretch is a great grounding posture that is made more challenging by your dog. It strengthens your legs, helps stability and opens the thoracic spine. You need to think about maintaining length throughout and having your dog on your hip reminds you to keep your torso stretched. He'll also help deepen the pose and actually make the pose harder as you really have to work with legs and core to support the extra weight.

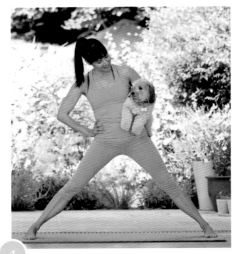

1 Start by standing with your feet wide apart, with your toes turned in slightly and your dog on your left hip.

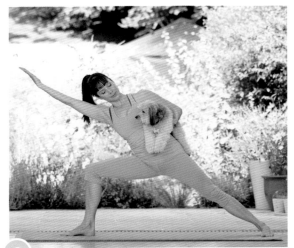

2 Turn your right foot out. Inhale and push out with your left leg, bending your right knee until it is above your right ankle bone. Extend your right arm out to the side, lengthening both sides of your waist, extending as fully as possible

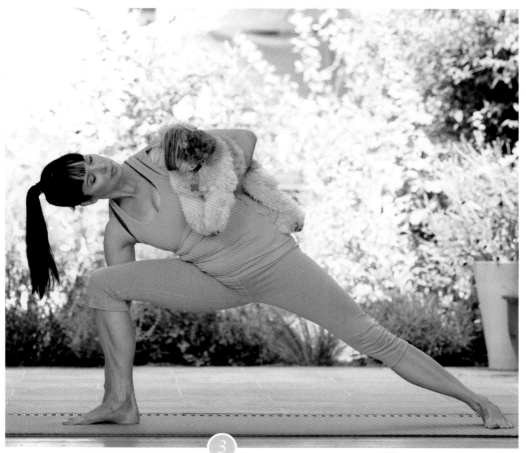

3 Maintaining eye contact as you move, exhale and place the right hand behind the right foot. Keep full extension. Inhale and rotate the navel towards the ceiling. As you do so your dog might move higher on your flank, which will help with the pressure on your knee. However, you can keep your dog on your hip in order to support him. To come back out of the pose, inhale and straighten the right leg. Once upright, release your dog or change sides if he's happy enough to continue.

Two-legged Friends

Squat Sequence with Dog Handstand ○
Malasana with Ardho Mukha Vrksasana

This is a position that involves both of you releasing your 'tired legs' after the strenuous standing poses in this chapter. In India, villagers squat naturally for hours, unlike us Westerners, who sit day in and day out on chairs, which weakens the back and upper back muscles. Squats are a healthy release for the lumbar region and naturally open the hips. This is also an opportunity for the Dogi to perform a Doga Handstand, which helps him eliminate tension in his back legs.

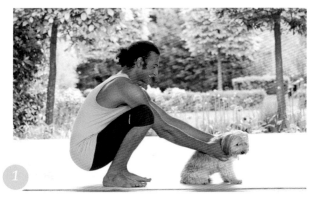

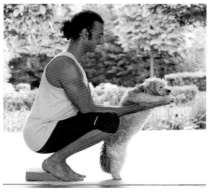

Come into a comfortable squat position, drawing your tail towards the ground, with your feet apart and your heels on the floor. Separate your knees and lean your torso forwards, bringing your upper arms between the knees.

Modification
If your heels don't touch the ground or if you suffer from bad knees and a weak lower back, place a block under your heels for support.

safety note 1
Consult a vet before practising this pose to the full extent, to be sure that your dog doesn't have any elbow abnormalities.

safety note 2
In these postures, it is important to observe Ahimsa and the principle of non-violence towards your dog (see pages 10 and 12).

Slide both hands under your dog's inner thigh, slightly tilt his pelvis forward, and lift both legs off the ground. His back legs will be lifted off the floor so all his weight will be distributed on his front legs. Slowly start massaging your dog, without too much pressure through the fingers, from the inner thigh to the outer thigh muscles and all the way around and up and down, drawing circular movements, again with not too much pressure. Avoid massaging the area about 2.5cm (1in) away from any joints, especially the tail. If your dog remains still in the posture and doesn't pull his legs away from you, you know you're doing a good job. Ensure that you put a little extra pressure through the glutes. This is where, like us humans, dogs are most tight. Massage for 3–5 minutes until both you and your dog want to come out of the pose.

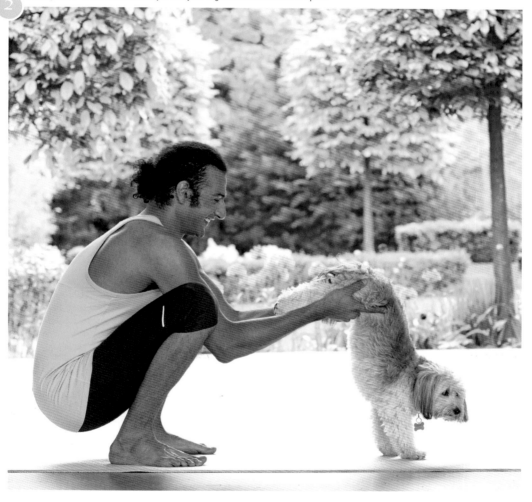

Get Into the Groove A

Standing Poses sequence

This sequence requires strength and flexibility – try it once you have mastered all the standing poses it contains. It's designed to build core strength, poise and stamina as well as the mental strength you will need to attempt more advanced poses later. A great rejuvenating sequence, it will make you break into a sweat!

*Downward Facing Dog
(Ardho Mukha Svanasana)*
Place your dog on the front of the mat and start from Downward Facing Dog.

Turn your left foot at a 75-degree angle, inhale and step your right leg forwards, keeping your left heel of the floor. Pick your dog up.

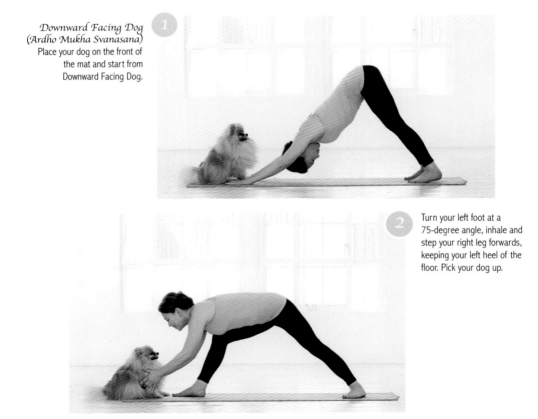

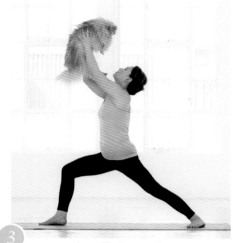

③ Warrior 1 (Virabhadrasana 1)
Inhale and lift your dog up in Warrior 1.

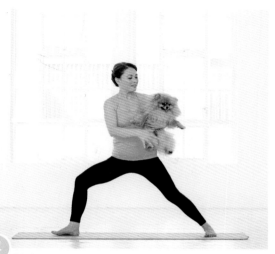

④ Exhale, lower your dog and place him on top of your upper left hip as you pivot your hips to the left.

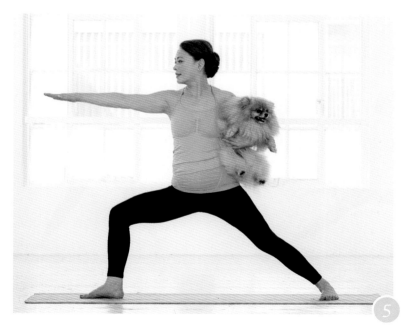

Warrior 11 (Virabhadrasana 11)
Inhale, extend your right arm out in line with your shoulders, gazing past the third finger, in Warrior 2. Stay in this pose for 3–5 breaths.

⑤

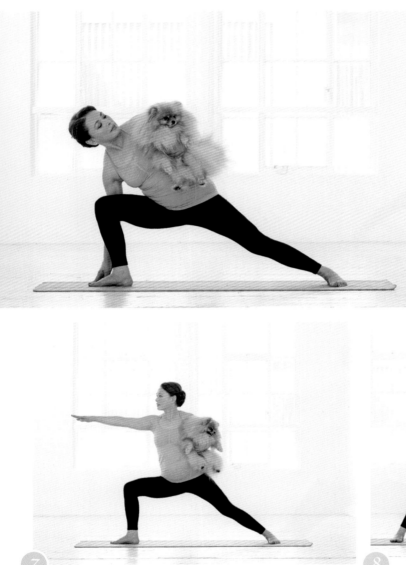

6

Extended side angle stretch (Uthita Parsvakonasana)
Exhale and place your right hand behind your right foot and extend both sides of the waistline, gazing at your dog and pressing into your left heel firmly. Stay in this pose for 3–5 breaths.

7

Warrior 2 (Virabhadrasana 2)
Inhale and come back up into Warrior 2.

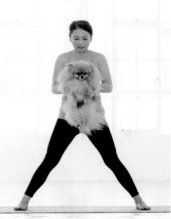

8

Straighten your right leg and exhale. Then move your dog over to your right hip to change sides.

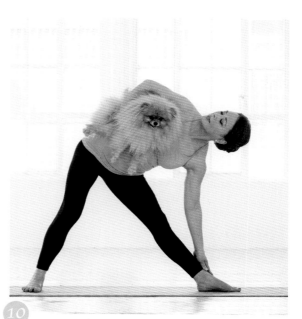

9 Inhale as you turn out your left foot at a 90-degree angle, and keep your rigth foot turned slightly inwards. Place your dog between your right hip and your waistline. Inhale and reach out with your left hand.

10 *Extended Triangle (Utthita Trikonasana)*
Exhale, place your left hand on your left ankle and turn to look over your right shoulder, keeping both legs strong and engaged. Stay in Extended Triangle Pose (left side) for 3–5 breaths. To release the pose, bend your left knee, inhale and come back up.

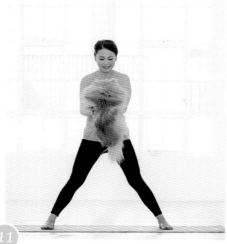

11 Exhale and stand with both feet parallel, holding your dog close to your chest. Continue breathing until your heart rate slows down.

12 *Wide-legged Forward Bend (Prasarita Padottanasana)*
Exhale and bend forwards from your waist, allowing the weight of your dog to draw you down. Now release your dog onto the mat and rest your hands and preferably your head on him to release the tension in your hips and neck. Stay in this pose for as long as you need to. To exit the pose, inhale and come up.

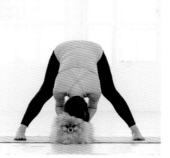

Get Into the Groove B

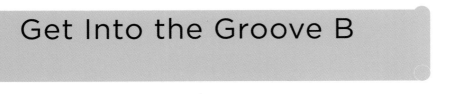

Intermediate Standing Poses sequence

Another sweat breaker, this sequence is a more advanced variation of Get into the Groove A, shown on the previous pages, with similar benefits. The transition from Warrior 2 on the right side into Warrior 2 on the left side requires a lot of strength through the ankles, thighs and quads. This sequence also opens the hips and shoulders and firms and tones the abdomen.

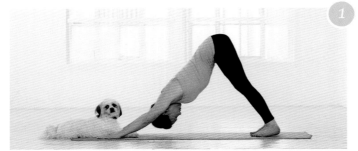

1 *Downward Facing Dog (Ardho Mukha Svanasana)*
Place your dog on the front of the mat and start in Downward Facing Dog. Hold for 3–5 breaths.

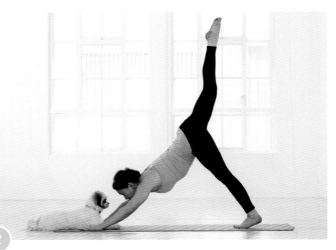

Inhale and extend your right leg up to the ceiling. **2**

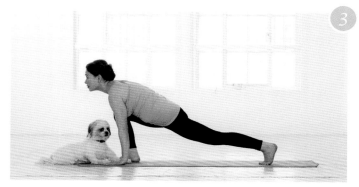

3. Runner's Lunge (Alanasana)

Exhale, swing your right leg through and lunge forwards, placing your right foot between both hands. Keep your back heel off the ground.

4. Warrior Lunge (Anjaneyasana)

Inhale and raise your dog above your head. Hold Warrior Lunge for 3–5 breaths.

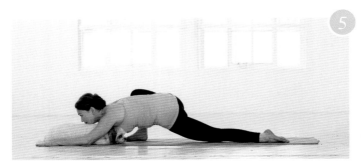

5 *Runner's Lunge (Alanasana)*
Exhale, bend forwards from your torso and place your dog on the mat. Place your hands on the mat and lower your left knee to the ground. Lower your forearms to the mat and stay in this pose for 3–5 breaths, resting your head on your dog.

6 Inhale, come up and pivot on your back foot, pressing into the outer heel. Pick up your dog and place him on your left hip.

Extended Side Angle Stretch (Uthita Parsvakonasana)
Inhale and extend your right arm out. Exhale, place your right hand behind your right foot, gaze at your dog and stay down in Hip Sitter for 3–5 breaths.

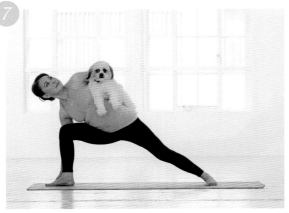

7

safety note

To avoid any lower back problems or other injuries, do not attempt this sequence if your dog weighs more than 5kg (11lb).

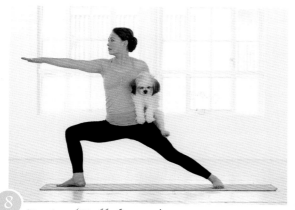

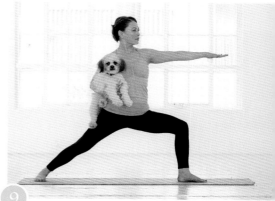

8 *Warrior 2 (Virabhadrasana 2)*
Inhale and lift up your torso, keeping your legs strong and firm. Exhale, extend the right arm, looking over your right finger and sink your hips into Warrior 2 on the right side. Hold for 3–5 breaths.

9 To swap sides, inhale and straighten your right leg. Reposition your feet, exhale and come down into Warrior 2 on the left side, extending your left arm out. Hold for 3–5 breaths.

10 Inhale, come back up and turn your feet parallel. Hold your dog close to your chest like a baby, so that he faces you, and make eye as you continue to breathe.

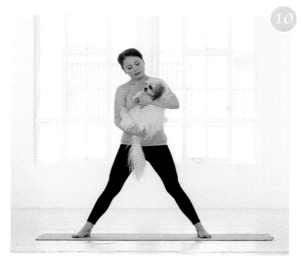

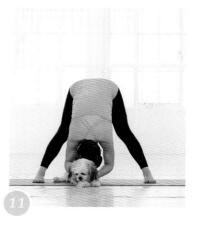

Wide-legged Forward Bend (Prasarita Padottanasana)
Exhale and bend forwards from your hips, letting the weight of your dog carry you into Wide-legged Forward Bend. Enjoy resting the crown of your head on your dog. Stay in this pose until you feel ready to come back up. Repeat the sequence on the left side. **11**

Seated yoga poses help you to train your spine to make it straight, strong and supple. It doesn't matter how far you can stretch – resistance in the body gives us the opportunity to learn and change. In time, through repetition, you will gain flexibility and a greater sense of calm.

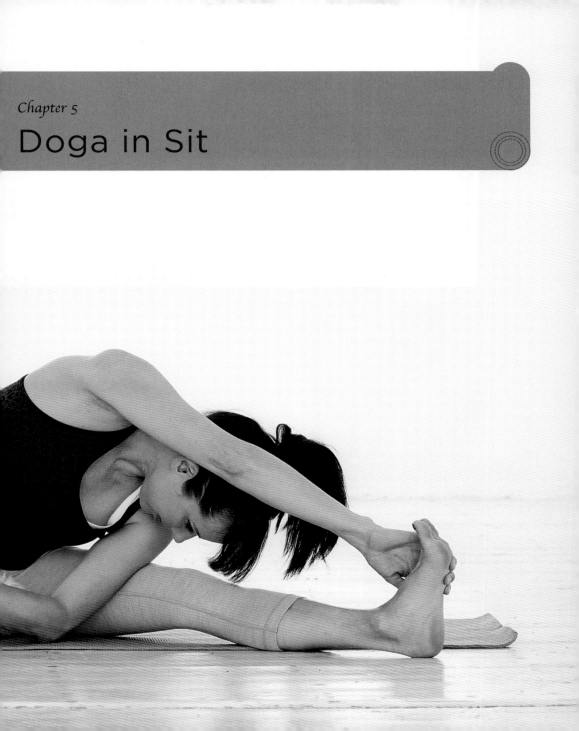

Chapter 5

Doga in Sit

The Hot Dog

Seated Forward Bend ○ *Paschimottanasana*

This pose helps stretch the legs and lower back, opening the backs of the legs and shoulders. It is a very emotional pose as you are bending forwards with your heart. This pose helps your dog to relax – it is perfect for anxious dogs – and I've also found that it aids their sleep and improves digestion.

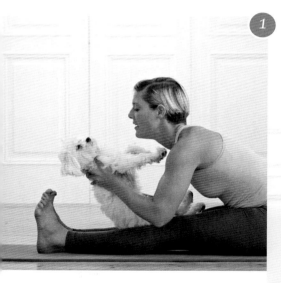

1 Sit on the floor with legs extended in front of you and your toes pointing upwards. Hold your dog in your arms, making eye contact and breathing. Inhale and press through your pelvis, keeping the front torso long, and lean forwards from the hip joints, not the waist.

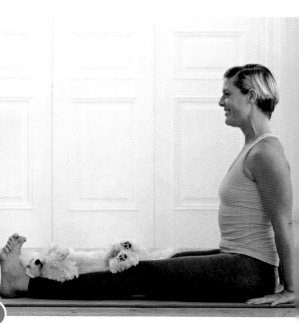

Settle your dog on your shins, lying on his back. Many dogs find this relaxing, but some feel vulnerable in this position, so switch him over to his front if you sense any anxiety. Sit back up straight.

2

Your dog will share your heart's rhythm in this yogic hug

As you reach forwards your head will be next to your dog's heart. Dogs in this pose will lose their fight-or-flight sensibilities and you'll engage their parasympathetic nervous system, slowing their heartbeat. You may find his heart will beat at the same pace as yours, making this the ultimate in bonding postures.

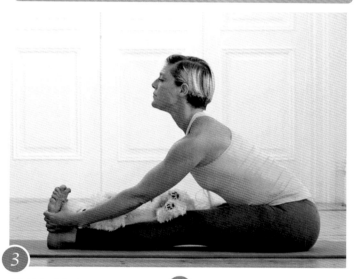

When he's calm and you're ready to go further, lengthen your tail bone, on an inhalation reach across your dog and hold your feet, with your elbows fully extended. If this isn't possible, you can always loop a strap around your feet to help you reach.

3

4

To extend the position further and make it even more of a bonding experience, exhale, collapse your elbows and lower your head to your dog's chest so you can hear his heartbeat. Breathe in time with his heartbeat to achieve unity.

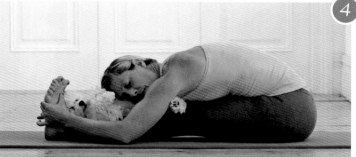

The Doggie Twister

Revolved Staff Pose ○ *Parivrtta Dandasana*

Revolved Staff Pose opens the outer hips, preparing you for later poses. Twisting poses are invigorating; they clear the mind and help release tension in your lower back and neck.

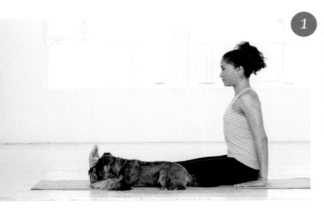

1 Begin with the Staff Pose: sit with your legs extended and your spine long. Place your dog slightly more in the direction of the upper left thigh, either lying on his belly or lying on his back in a supine position. Make sure he is comfortable and massage him until he's settled. Press your hands into the ground next to your hips without lifting your sitting bones off the floor. Drop your chin towards the sternum and create a Victorious Breathing sound (see page 24).

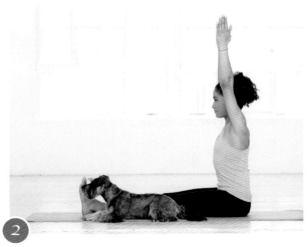

On an inhale, raise your arms over your head and bring your palms to face each other. Lift your chest and draw your shoulders away from the ears. **2**

3 Begin the twist on an exhale. As you turn through your torso, extend your legs and flex your toes. Reach your righ hand across your legs to the outside of the left knee. Rest your left palm on your dog. Bring your left hand to the ground behind your left hip. Look over your left shoulder. Breathe deeply into the twist and keep massaging your dog. On an exhale, unfold the twist and return to Step 1. Repeat on the right side, remembering to move your dog over to your other side.

The Surfer

Upward Plank Pose ○ *Purvattanasana*

This intense stretch is the counterpose to the postures on pages 74–5. Doing this pose restores balance in the body, strengthens and tones the abdomen, legs and arms, and prepares you for more strenuous poses. Your dog becomes your 'buddy' by simply sitting or standing on your hips like a surfer. His weight reminds you of the muscles you need to engage to maintain stability and lightness as you would on a surfboard. Dogs have an amazing sense of balance; you needn't worry about your dog's core strength – instead, focus on yours. Your dog may jump off a few times and that's fine. Practice makes perfect.

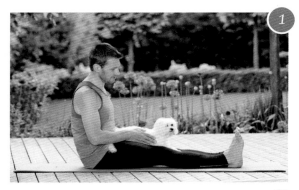

1. Sit upright in Staff Pose with your feet hip-distance apart. Keep your legs engaged and toes flexed. Place your dog on your upper thighs lying flat on his belly, either facing towards you or away from you. Steady your dog with soothing strokes from top to tail.

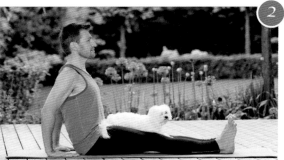

2. Exhale and take your hands about 20cm (8in) behind your buttocks. Place them down flat on the mat and shoulder-distance apart.

Continue to exhale, drawing the shoulder blades together. On an inhale, lift up your hips, extending your tailbone forwards. Press the weight of your body evenly through both hands and feet. Keep your abdomen strong and engaged to maintain the perfect surfboard for your dog. Hold for 3–5 breaths. If you have a tight neck, avoid taking your head back. Keep your chin in line with your sternum to maintain stability throughout. Exhale and slowly lower yourself down to Step 1.

3

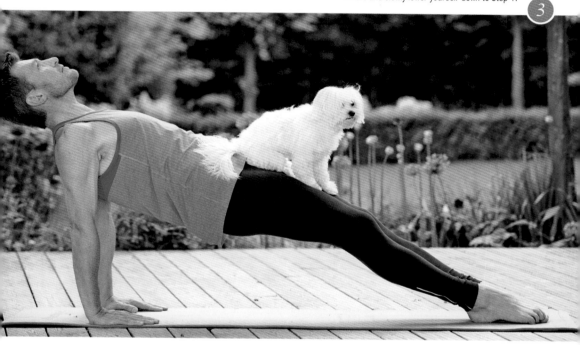

Modification
Instead of keeping your legs straight, bend your knees and place your feet flat on the ground. Exhale and press up firmly and evenly through both feet into Reverse Table Pose.

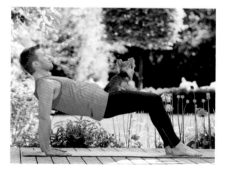

counterpose
Bend forwards from your hips to stretch out your lower back muscles (See pages 74–5).

The Twisted Sage

Seated Spinal Twist ○ *Marichyasana*

Spinal twists are very effective: they rejuvenate and invigorate the spinal column, stimulate the brain and also massage the abdominal organs, including the kidneys and liver. These poses open the breath and help you to deepen and lengthen the exhalation, which helps your dog to relax.

1 Sit upright in Staff Pose, bend your right knee and put your right foot on the floor in line with your right buttock. Make sure your dog is next to your right hip. Place your right hand on his back and massage his neck for reassurance. Keep your left leg strong and slightly rotated inwards.

On an inhale, extend your left arm up. With an exhalation, rotate your torso towards the outer right thigh. Maintain length in both sides of the waist. Keep exhaling and twisting until you manage to hook your left upper arm over your outer right knee. Now try to release your left hand onto your dog. **2**

This twisting pose is named after the sage Marichi, the son of Brahma

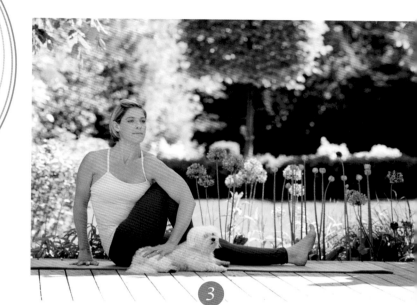

3

Inhale and swing your right hand behind your right buttock, lifting through the sternum and drawing your shoulder blades down and away from your ears so you maintain length through the spine. Look over your right shoulder. Keep breathing evenly through the nose. With your left hand, continue to massage or stroke your dog. Hold the twist for as long as comfortable.

Modification

For beginners, keep your right hand on your dog and twist only as far as is comfortable, flexing your left hand.

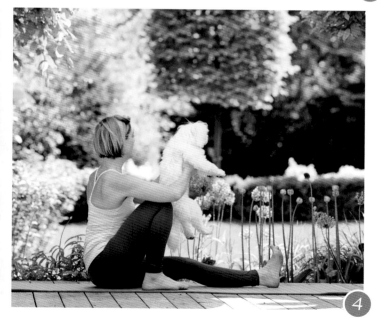

4

On an exhalation, unfold the twist and return to Staff Pose. Move your dog over to the other side and repeat on the left.

The Samurai

Hero ○ *Virasana*

This pose lets you meditate on your breathing practice. Sitting in this pose reminds me of a Samurai but, instead of going to war, the Yogi contemplates his or her inner battle with the ego. Ask yourself the questions on the right, then use some of the breathing exercises from Chapter 2 to rest the mind and connect with your dog. Child's Pose (See pages 44–5) is a great counterpose to the Hero.

○ Has my mind wandered off into the future or the past?
○ How is my dog doing in this moment?
○ Am I fully present and awake in this moment?
○ Am I expecting perfection of my dog and myself?

1 Kneel on the floor with your knees together. Separate your feet so that they are wider than your hips and bring your seat to the floor. If this is impossible, slide a cushion or a yoga block under your sitting bones. Place your dog on top of your thighs, keeping the thighs firm and rolled inwards. Become still and strong like a Samurai. Breathing deeply and gently, place both hands, palms soft and flat, on your dog's lower ribs. Can you feel his diaphragm expanding and contracting? Can you help your dog's heart rate slow down? Imagine you were able to breathe together in unison.

2 Place your dog on your thighs, either facing towards you or away from you. Perform 3–5 rounds of sharp Lion Breaths (See page 25), then regulate your breathing by breathing through your nose.

Modification
If you have bad knees or tight hips, tuck your toes under, for lumbar support.

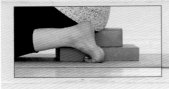

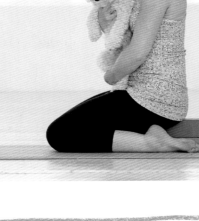

Rolling Down the River

The Boat ○ Navasana

'Nava' means 'boat', so imagine you and your dog floating down a river. You are the boat and your dog is the captain, reminding you to stay steady and strong. This pose strengthens the lower back and abdomen.

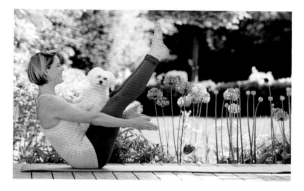

Large Boat Pose

Sit on your mat, with your legs extended in front of you. Place your dog on your upper thighs, lying on his back. If he's reluctant to lie back, place him on your shins instead. Lift your legs up and sit squarely on your buttocks. Straighten your back and legs to create the V-shaped keel. Lift your chest and draw in your abdomen wall in. Breathe deeply on the exhalation. Lock your anus muscles. Straighten your arms to the side of your knees. Try not to collapse in your lower back or chest. Stay in this pose for as long as is comfortable, but avoid straining the breath.

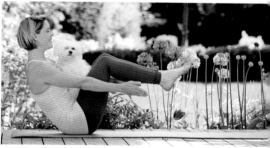

Modification: Little Boat Pose

If you are a beginner or you have a smaller or a restless dog, place him on your knees or shins facing you. Perform the posture with your bent knees. Avoid hunching the shoulders; instead, draw your shoulders away from the ears.

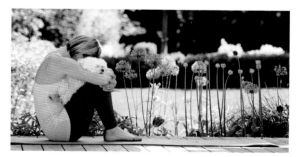

Counterpose

This forward bend is a counterpose to the Boat. Draw your knees towards the chest and wrap your arms around your knees. Keep a soft curvature in your lower back. If you dog has been sitting on your thighs, you may want to include him in this pose. But be careful not to squash your dog as you bring your knees in to the chest. If he wants to jump off, let him go and have a sniff around.

The Pancake

Wide-angle Seated Bend ○ *Upavistha Konasana*

This symmetrical deep forward bend stretches the insides and backs of the legs. It deeply releases the groin and strengthens the spine. In this posture, your dog can relax, possibly even take a nice snooze, and enjoy your presence and your Doga practice without needing to be active. Your dog can either lie on this back or flat on his front paws, whichever he seems to prefer.

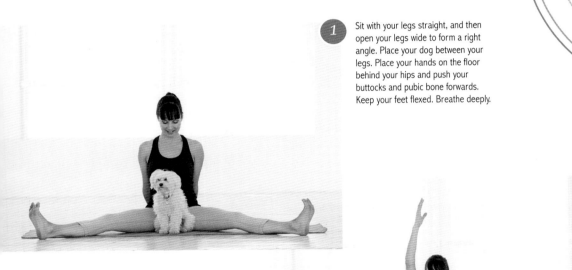

1 Sit with your legs straight, and then open your legs wide to form a right angle. Place your dog between your legs. Place your hands on the floor behind your hips and push your buttocks and pubic bone forwards. Keep your feet flexed. Breathe deeply.

2 On an inhale, place your left hand on your dog and extend both sides of your waist as you extend your right arm straight up.

3 On an exhale, reach over with your right hand to catch the outer edge of your left foot. Keep your feet firmly flexed. On an inhale, rotate your navel up towards the ceiling and rotate your head so you can gaze under your right shoulder. If this creates too much pressure on your neck, look down at the floor. Hold for 3—5 breaths.

To come out of the posture, exhale and lengthen both sides of your waist. As you inhale, lift up through your chest and come back up into the sitting position in Step 1.

Modification
If you can't catch your foot, bend your knees.

While you stretch and strengthen your body, your dog can relax

counter-release

To counter-release the Wide-angle Seated Bend, slowly walk your hands forwards and bring the front of your torso down onto your dog. If you have difficulty bending that far forwards, bend your knees slightly. Release the neck and breathe deeply.

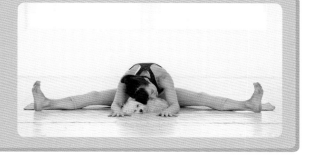

The Sailor

Both Big Toe Pose ◯ *Ubhaya Padangusthasana*

This is a very challenging pose, similar to The Boat (See page 83). As before, your dog is a reminder of how hard your abdomen needs to work in order for you to stay afloat. Only this time the V-shape is tighter: you must find the ultimate pivotal point in your sitting bones in which you can catch your toes and extend the legs at the same time without collapsing in the lower back or chest. In this posture your dog is once more your passenger, once more you can reassure him that you are capable of being the leader. You are in charge of transferring your stillness to your dog, so make the most of it.

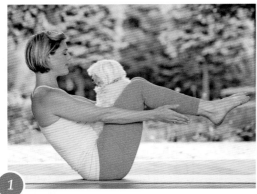

Sit in Little Boat Pose with bent knees, with your dog placed on your thighs.

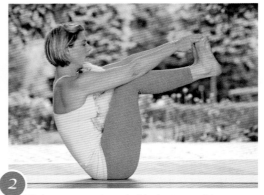

Exhale, curve your spine and roll back onto your sitting bones. Engage your abdomen and catch both toes. Inhale and extend both legs equally; keep your toes firmly pointed.

Continue to inhale and straighten the
lower back as you open your chest.
Exhale and take your head back.
See if you can stay balanced in this
pose for a few deep breaths.

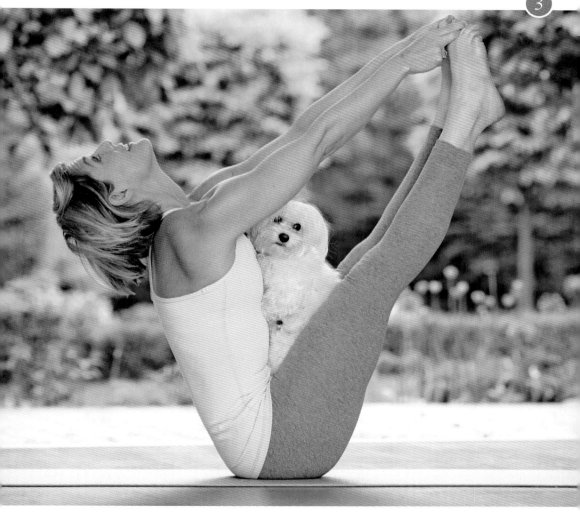

Sail Away

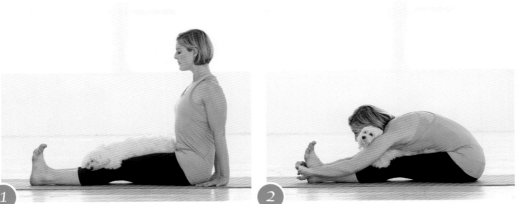

Seated Poses sequence

Sail Away is a fun sequence that takes you through folds, bends and twists. It's also one of the easier sequences to master. Think of it like an adventurous journey down a river, complete with a camel ride for your dog! Poses such as The Boat and Upward Plank help you strengthen the muscles around the mid and lower spine and develop your overall core strength, while the Seated Spinal Twist is a nice counterpose in between, to help you to neutralize your spine and draw your senses inwards. The sequence ends with a more challenging posture, the Camel (See pages 114–15), which you can gradually work your way towards achieving – it can take a little time and repetition. Please practise this sequence on an empty stomach.

1

Staff Pose (Dandasana)
Sit in Staff Pose with a straight spine, hands resting next to your sides, with your dog resting on your upper thighs, facing away from you.

2

Seated Forward Bend (Paschimottanasana)
Exhale and fold forwards from your hip crease and rest your chest on your dog. Stay for 3–5 breaths in Seated Forward Bend.

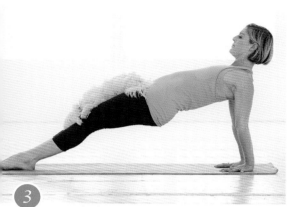

3 Upward Plank (Purvattanasana)

Place your hands 8–10cm (3–4in) behind your sitting bones. Inhale and lift your hips up towards the ceiling. Exhale and take your head back or, if you have a tight neck, keep your chin towards your chest. Hold Upward Plank for 3–5 breaths, then come back down on an exhale.

4 Seated Spinal Twist (Marichyasana)

Place your dog on the outside of your left sitting bone. Bend your left knee, keeping the left heel in line with your left sitting bone. Exhale and twist your torso to the left. Inhale and swing your left hand behind your sitting bones, resting your right hand on your dog. Look over your left shoulder and down your nose. Stay in Seated Spinal Twist for 3–5 breaths then exhale and undo the twist.

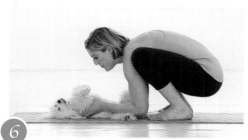

5 The Boat (Navasana)

Place your dog on the top of your thigh bones, so he sits on his back legs facing you. (If he is a larger dog he'll be resting his paws on your chest.) Inhale and raise both legs off the ground so they are extended out with toes pointed. Extend your arms forwards, turning the palms of your hands inwards and drawing your shoulders blades down towards the mid-spine. Hold The Boat for 3–5 breaths.

6 Squat Pose (Malasana)

Exhale, place both feet on the ground and roll your weight forwards onto the balls of your feet. Stay in Squat Pose, resting your dog on the floor, between your legs, with both hands on his belly. Give him a nice belly massage while you soften and ease out your hips in this counterpose.

*Reclining Hero
pose stretches the
muscles on the front
of your body*

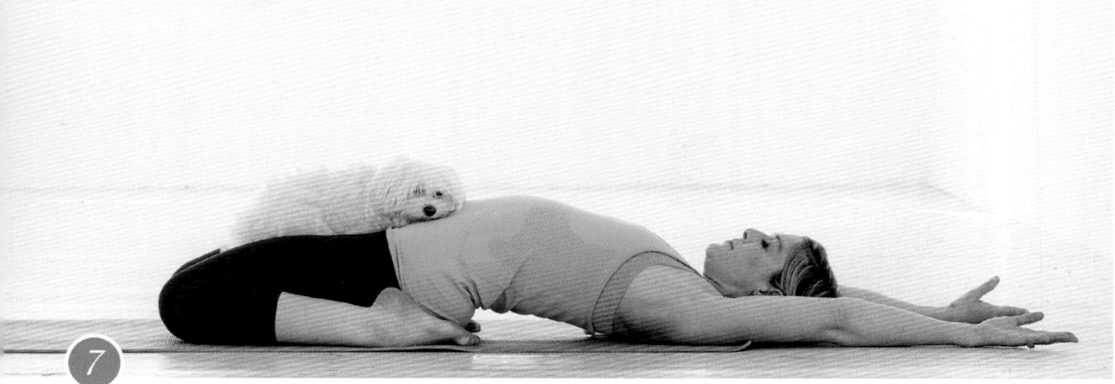

⑦

Reclining Hero (Supta Virasana)

Exhale and kneel on the floor with your knees together. To come into Reclining Hero pose, separate your feet so that they are wider than your hips and bring your seat to the floor. Place your dog on top of your thighs, keeping the thighs firm and rolled inwards. Let go of your dog and place your hands on the floor beside your hips. Exhale and lower yourself down backwards onto your forearms then if you are comfortable, continue lowering your back towards the floor. Inhale and reach your arms over your head. Keep your thighs firmly engaged and breathe deeply into your abdomen so your dog can feel your breath. Stay in Reclining Hero for 3–5 breaths, then slowly come back up.

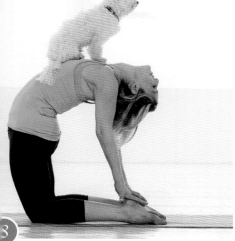

Camel (Ustrasana)

Come onto your knees in preparation for The Camel. With the help of a Doga buddy, place your dog on your chest. Inhale and lift through your chest. Exhale and reach your hands back to take hold of your heels. Stay for 3–5 breaths, breathing deeply into your chest. Inhale and come back up again. You'll need your Doga buddy to take your dog off your chest before you come up.

Child's Pose (Balanasana)

Exhale and sit back, resting on your heels. Lean forwards from your torso and rest the front of your chest on your dog. Stay in Child's Pose for as long as you need to. Breathe deeply from your abdomen and connect with your dog's heartbeat.

The Half Hot Dog

Three-limbed forward bend ○
Tiriang Mukha Eka Pada Paschimottanasana

Like the Hot Dog Pose on pages 74–5, this posture focuses on the unique and natural bond we have with our dogs. As you lay your chest flat on your dog's chest, he will be able to feel your heartbeat and vice versa. This posture facilitates the inward rotation of the hip joint. It creates flexibility in the knee joint and also improves digestion.

1 From Staff Pose, fold your left leg back at the knee. Roll the calf muscles out to the side to allow your outer left thigh to drop towards the floor without catching on the calf. There should be no discomfort in the knee joint. If necessary, sit on a folded blanket or yoga block until the knee can close more deeply. Place your dog along the inside of your right calf — either lying back or flat on his stomach. Massage your dog until he feels ready to submit. Now let go and sit upright.

2 Inhale and extend your spine out of your pelvis and reach forwards with your right hand to take hold of your right foot. (Bend your right knee if you can't reach.) Open up and lift your chest away from your right leg. Square your shoulders and sit down into your left buttock so that the hips are square.

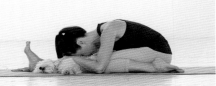

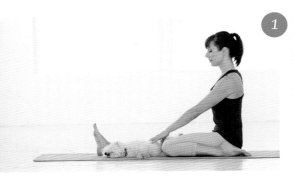

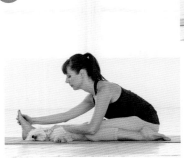

3 Exhale, bend from your hips and fold your torso forwards over your right leg, releasing your hand flat to the floor. If you can, get your head to touch your dog. Breathe deeply through the chest and abdomen and stay in this pose for as long as it is comfortable.

observation

Try resting your head on your dog, if you can: this not only connects your nervous systems but also helps to slow down the heart rate.

modifications

Depending on the size of your dog, you may have to experiment a little with placement. A small, light dog, such as a chihuahua, may be happy to sit on top of your right upper thigh while you bend forwards from your hips. A larger, heavier dog will need a little more space to stretch out, so try placing him on the inside of your leg, as shown here.

 Inhale and lift from the chest as you extend your torso forwards, then exhale and come back up into Staff Pose. Repeat on the other side.

Pigeon on Dog Pose

One-legged King Pigeon Pose ○ *Eka Pada Rajakapotasana*

The One-legged King Pigeon pose is a powerful hip opener, stretching the muscles of the external hip rotators of the bent front leg and the groin of the extended back leg. It is important to make sure that your hips are open in this pose, to avoid any compression in the lower back. The more you relax into this pose, the more you release tension and emotions stored in your hips – this release can be quite an intense sensation.

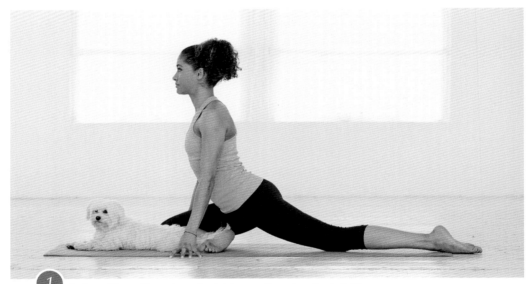

1 Begin on all fours, with your knees directly below your hips and your hands slightly ahead of your shoulders. Bring your right knee forwards so that it rests behind your right wrist and angle your shin under your torso, so that your right foot is to the front of your left knee. The outside of your right shin will now rest on the floor. Slowly slide your left leg back – keep pointing your toes so that you can feel the full extension of your back leg straightening. Now lower the front of the left thigh and the outside of your right buttock towards the floor.

On an exhale, slowly walk your hands forwards. The right leg will stretch the psoas muscles and other hip flexors. Lengthening through the front of your torso, go as deep into this forward bend as you can, but without straining your knee or lower back. If you fancy stretching out your tight neck muscles, rest your chest and head on your dog and turn your head on each side for 5 breaths. Stay in this posture for as long as you want to, but ensure that you and your dog remain comfortable.

On an inhale, press down into the floor, extend the lower back and lengthen your waistline. Lift from your sternum and keep pointing your left foot as you slowly return to Step 1 on an exhalation. Release and relax into Seated Forward Bend before repeating the posture on the left side.

*Challenging
but restorative,
this pose opens
your hips, chest
and shoulders*

Modification

If you have a weak lower back, wedge a block under your left upper thigh, to avoid compression in the lumbar spine. Roll the upper left hip slightly forwards and draw your right sitting bone back. Try and press your left thigh down into the block.

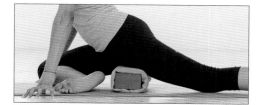

These postures and sequences build up core strength by incorporating weight-bearing poses, backbends and poses that engage the lower abdomen. For your dog, these are trust exercises, with your strength being his stability, while his weight on you is your mental challenge.

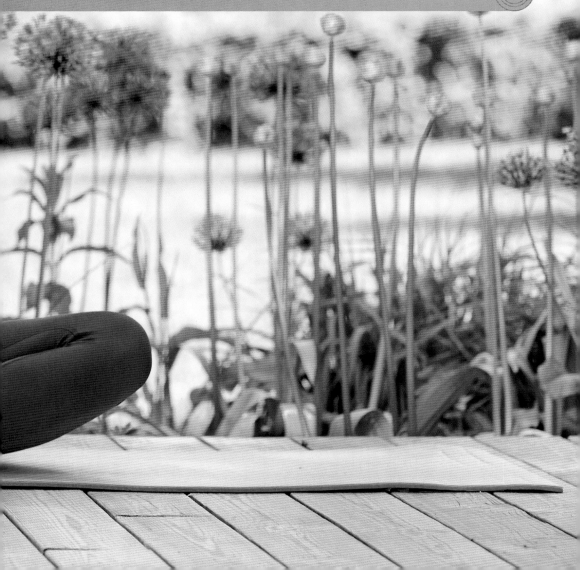

Chapter 6

Strong to the Core

Walk the Plank

Downward Dog Plank Variation ○
Adho Mukha Svanasana and Utthita Chaturanga Dandasana

This sequence is a great way to strengthen the upper body and prepare for some more advanced postures. Your dog's weight on your lower back will remind you to remain stable in the sacrum and strong in the abdomen. Your dog will need to trust you completely, so this pose is excellent for building confidence and calm in your dog. A nice counterpose to this sequence is the Child's Pose (See pages 44–5).

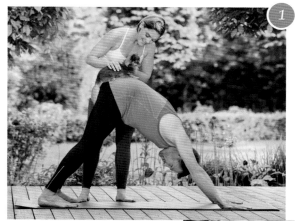

1 Come into Downward Facing Dog. Allow your Doga buddy to place your dog on your sacrum bone, lying flat on his belly in the direction of your head.

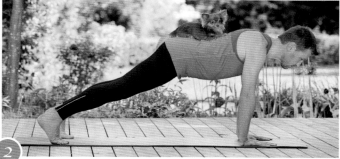

On an exhalation, draw your torso forwards until your arms are perpendicular to the floor and your shoulders are directly over your wrists. To keep your dog remaining seated on your back, you must engage the quads and press firmly into your toes. Avoid collapsing in the lower back. Stay in this pose for 3–5 breaths and continue holding the pose, even if your dog jumps off. *2*

gently does it

Some dogs are happy to be seated at a higher level than usual, while others panic when they lose contact with, or can't see, the floor. Each dog reacts differently. It is therefore important to cultivate patience and an attitude of non-violence (See page 12). If your dog refuses to do the pose or is scared, don't push him.

3 To return to Downward Facing Dog, inhale and draw your shoulder blades apart and up through your navel as you continue to lift through your sitting bones, shifting the weight back into your legs. Keep your head and neck relaxed. When you return to Downward Facing Dog, get your Doga buddy to place your dog on the floor.

Dog on Cat Pose

Cat Stretch ⟳ *Marjaryasana*

The Cat Stretch is famous for its therapeutic benefits as you explore the natural curvatures of the spine. It also provides a gentle massage for the muscles between and around the vertebra. The weight of your dog on top of your sacrum bone makes this posture a lot more challenging, but also connects you with the more deep-seated muscles of your lower back. This pose works both ways: your dog receives a gentle massage under his belly as you flex and extend the spine while you, in return, receive a stretch by him sitting on top of your back.

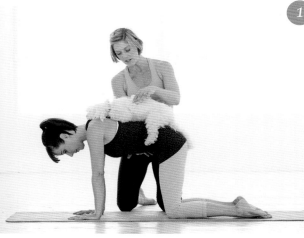

1 Start on your hands and knees with your lower back in a 'table-top' position (imagine your lower back is as a flat table). Allow your Doga buddy to place your dog on top of your table with your dog lying flat on his stomach facing in the same direction as you. Make sure your knees are set directly below your hips and your wrists, elbows and shoulders are in line and perpendicular to the floor, with your eyes looking at the floor.

As you exhale, round your spine towards the ceiling like a 'hissing cat'. You may want your Doga buddy to place a hand on your dog so he doesn't slip off. Release your head towards the floor and draw your chin slightly towards the chest. Inhale, coming back to the 'table-top' position on your hands and knees. Repeat these two movements several times. **2**

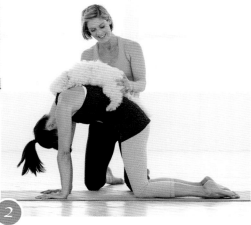

*You will need
a Doga buddy
to help you
with this pose*

When you are ready, rest in
Child's Pose, perhaps with your
dog still sitting on top.

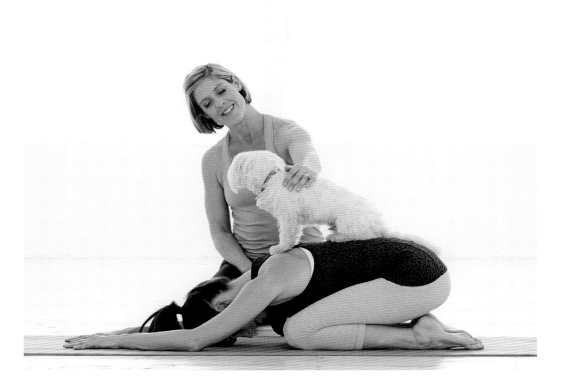

The Wood Chopper

Standing Forward Bend with Interlaced Hands ○ *Uttanasana*

The Woodchopper is the same pose as the Standing Forward Bend (See page 29), but this time the fingers are interlaced behind the back and your dog is sitting on your sacrum bone. To perform this pose, you require a Doga buddy. This posture stretches out lower back muscles, tight hamstrings, ankles and neck. In this posture you're bringing your whole weight through the front of the torso, making this an intense flexion. Your dog aids as a weight/prop and helps to stretch out your lower back muscles. This posture builds up trust and enhances your natural bond with your dog.

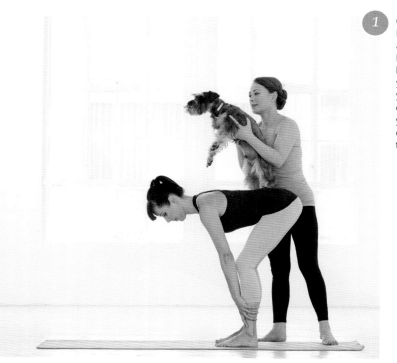

1 Come into Standing Forward Bend, with feet hip-distance apart and knees slightly bent. Keep a flat back so your Doga buddy can place your dog on your sacrum bone. Ensure your dog is comfortable. On an exhalation, bend forwards from your hips and grab hold of your calves. Keep your Doga buddy there for support.

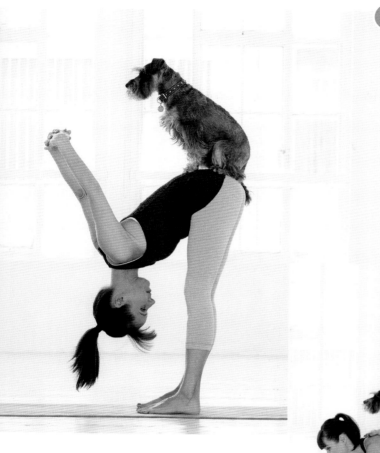

 Slide your hands down your calves and fold into your body like a deckchair. If you feel comfortable, stretch your arms up behind your back and interlock your fingers. Hold for 3–5 breaths.

Lower your arms, unlace your fingers and slide your hands back down to your calves. Bend your knees slightly. Inhale and extend your spine into Half Forward Bend. Get your Doga buddy to place your dog down on the floor. Continue to inhale as you come up into Mountain Pose.

Taking Off

Warrior 3 ○ *Virabhadrasana 3*

One of the more strengthening of the balancing poses, Warrior 3 also brings harmony and poise into your practice. With the help of a Doga buddy, you and your dog can enjoy 'taking off', you being the aeroplane and the dog, the passenger. Dogs usually enjoy balancing-on-all-fours poses, but should your dog feel uncomfortable, allow him to jump off. This pose may take several attempts to perfect, so be patient. Having your dog on top reminds you to keep your abdomen strong. This pose helps your dog to gain confidence and trust in you. To counterpose this posture, come into Seated Forward Bend (See pages 74–5).

Start in Mountain Pose with your feet hip-distance apart. Bend forwards from your hip crease, keeping your back long and straight. Catch your knees if you're tight in the hips. Inhale and extend your lower back to create a flat surface for your dog to sit on. Get your Doga buddy to place your dog on your lower back. (With a heavier dog, you will need to curve your spine slightly, so he doesn't slip off.) Press your feet firmly into the ground and lift up from your kneecaps to engage the upper thighs.

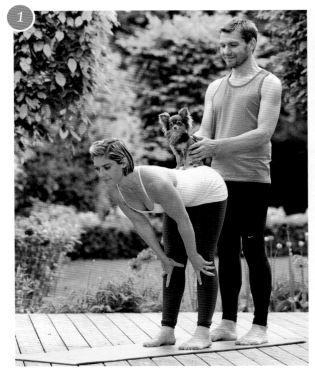

Exhale and bend your right knee as you bring more weight onto the right foot and raise the left leg. Inhale and straighten the right knee and foot, and lift your arms out to the sides, like an aeroplane, keeping them firm and outstretched. Try to lean as far forward as you can so your navel is stacked over your right foot. Breathe deeply and stay for as long as you can hold the posture. Use your Doga buddy for support. After several breaths, exhale and return to Half Forward Bend so your Doga buddy can take your dog off your back. Let him have a little wander around before you try the left side.

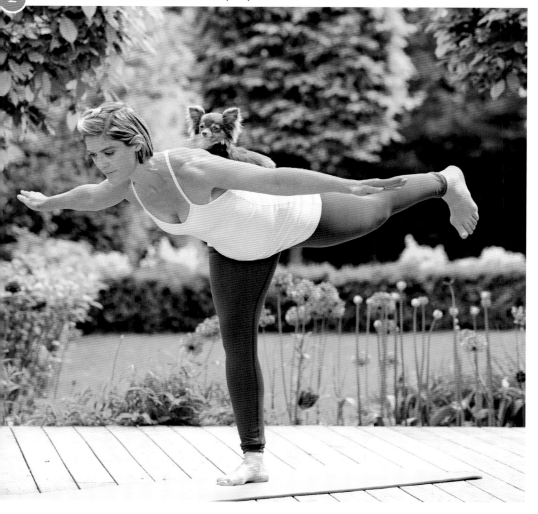

Dog meets Pigeon and Rides a Camel

Hip flexor sequence

Designed to work the hip flexors, this sequence builds up the strength and flexibiliy needed to master the peak posture – the Camel (See pages 114–15). Practice this sequence on an empty stomach, preferably in the morning.

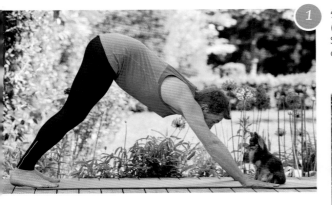

1 *Downward Facing Dog (Adho Mukha Svanasa)*
Start from Downward Facing Dog with your dog on the front of the mat.

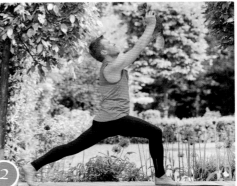

Warrior 1 (Virabhadrasana 1)
Exhale and step through with your right foot into Warrior Lunge. Pick your dog up off the floor and, on an inhale, lift him up over your head. Hold for 3–5 breaths. **2**

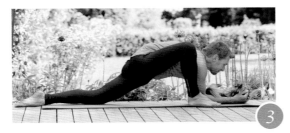

Runner's Lunge (Alanasana)
Exhale and lunge forwards into Runner's Lunge, resting your dog on his back on the inside of your foot. **3**

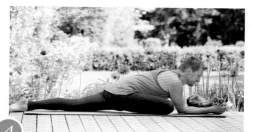

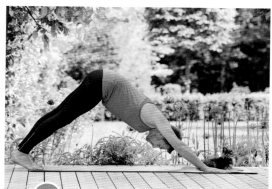

4 Pigeon
(Eka Pada Rajakapotasana)
Inhale, bring your right shin down and in line with the front of the mat and extend your left leg back, pointing your toes. Exhale, fold forwards from hips and bend forwards as far as you can in Pigeon Pose. Hold for 8–10 breaths, either massaging your dog with one hand or resting the dog on the inside of your forearm. (To gain more flexibility, lower yourself onto your elbows.)

5 Downward Facing Dog
(Adho Mukha Svanasa)
Rest your dog on the mat and inhale. Swing your right leg back into Downward Facing Dog and take 5–8 breaths in this pose.

6 Camel (Ustrasana)
Exhale, bring your knees to the floor and place both your hands at your waist. Ask your Doga buddy to place your dog on your chest. Inhale and lift your sternum. Exhale, bend backwards and grab hold of your heels. Stay in Camel for 3–5 breaths. Allow your dog to jump off your chest before you inhale and come back up.

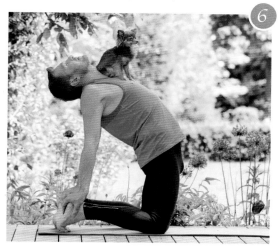

Child's Pose (Balasana)
Place your dog at the front of your mat, exhale and sit back onto your heels. Rest in Child's Pose, making eye contact with your dog.

7
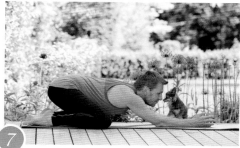

Strong as a Hero and Light as a Crow

Hip-opening sequence ○

This sequence has a hip-opening theme, followed by stretches that prepare you for 'taking flight' in The Crow (See pages 112–13), a more advanced pose. Don't despair if you struggle with this forearm balance at first – with dedication and practice you'll be as light as a crow.

1

Wide-legged Forward Bend (Upavistha Konasana)

On an inhale, reach up through your left hand, placing your right hand on your dog. Extend both sides of your waist as you reach with your left hand to catch the outer edge of your right foot. Stay in Wide-legged Forward Bend for 3–5 breaths.

2 Inhale, reach back up and exhale. Repeat the same movement on the other side, keeping eye contact with your dog.

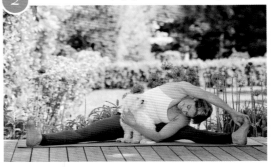

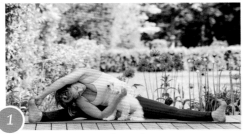

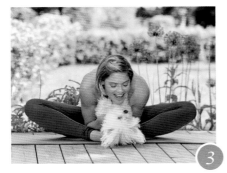

Cobbler's Pose (Baddha Konasana)

Exhale and bring the soles of the feet together. Pull your heels towards your pelvis and rotate your feet so the soles face the ceiling. Roll your hips back and place your dog on your feet. Exhale and bend forwards from your torso, bringing your chest onto your dog. Stay here for 5–8 breaths.

3

relax

Once you have completed this sequence, rest in Child's Pose (See pages 44–5) to release your lower back for a few breaths.

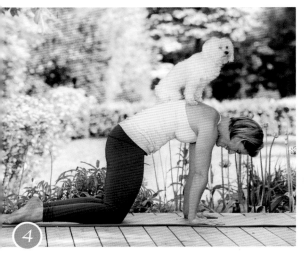

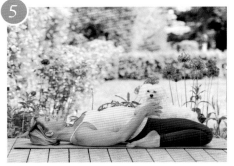

Reclining Hero (Supta Virasana)

To open your hips for Reclined Hero, exhale and sit back on your knees, rolling the thighs inwards. Continuing to exhale, place your dog on your upper thighs and lean back, resting first on your hands, then on your forearms, until you're fully in Reclined Hero. Hold for 5 breaths. Walk your hands back in and come up when you have had enough.

Cat Stretch (Marjaryasana)

Place your dog on the floor. Come onto your hands and knees for Cat Stretch. Ask a Doga buddy to place your dog on your back. Inhale, round your upper back and exhale, extending your tail towards the back of the room. Repeat the Cat Stretch for as long as your dog feels comfortable.

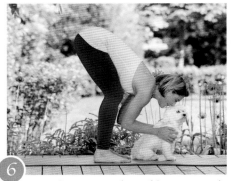

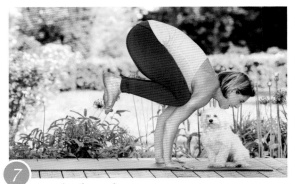

Standing Forward Bend (Uttanasana)

As a counterpose come into Standing Forward Bend. Stay in this pose until you've had enough, massaging your dog and making eye contact with him. Exhale, bend your knees even more and shift your weight onto the front balls of your feet.

Crow (Bakasana)

Place your dog at the front of your mat for a focus point. Place both hands on the floor. Bend the elbows and lean your shins on the back of your upper arms, making a shelf for your shins to sit on. Inhale and look forwards into your dog's eyes, raising the sitting bones and heels off the floor. Stay in Crow for 3–5 breaths.

These challenging postures require strength and flexibility. When you master a peak pose, you will feel a deep sense of accomplishment, freedom and empowerment. Your Dogi will sense your delight and both of you can experience being on top of the world.

Chapter 7

Top Dogi: Advanced Poses

Dog Kisses Crow

The Crow ○ *Bakasana*

The Crow Pose takes a little courage. But there's nothing to worry about because your dog will be there at the front of your mat as a mental block stopping you from worrying that you might fall over. You might even get distracted while he licks your face. This posture strengthens the upper back, arms and wrists and massages your inner organs. A steady gaze and strong regular Victorious Breathing (See page 24) is required to maintain poise, strength and concentration. For your dog it's a great opportunity to become curious about your breathing and to witness your 'inner calm'.

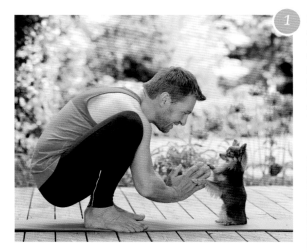

1 Place your dog at the front of the mat, ensuring that he faces you. (You may have to hold a treat between your teeth, just this once.) Come into a comfortable squat position, drawing your tail towards the ground, with your feet apart and the heels on the floor. Separate the knees and lean your torso forwards, bringing the upper arms between the knees.

Bring your palms to the floor and spread out the fingers. Bend your elbows and lean your shins on the backs of the upper arms, making a shelf for the shins to sit on.

2

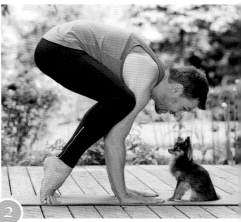

see the funny side

Don't forget to enjoy yourself! It's important to maintain a sense of humour during your Doga practice. If you lose your balance, start to wobble or fall over, don't worry – it happens to everyone. Just smile and try again. It's all about practice and progress, not perfection.

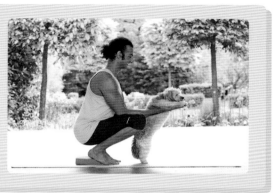

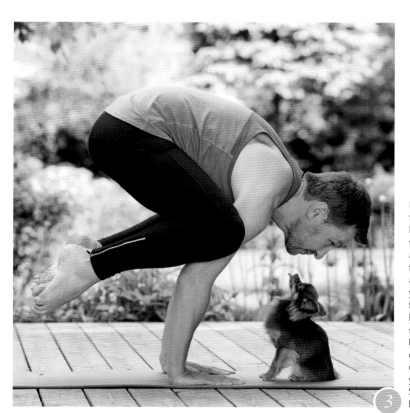

Inhale and look forwards, raising the seat and heels, and begin bending the elbows, bringing the weight onto the backs of your arms. Exhale and lift your weight forwards so that the shoulders are stacked over the wrists and your feet begin to lift off the floor, either one foot at a time or both feet together. Once you feel steady, bring your inner ankle bones together and lift your feet closer to the buttocks. Smile and don't forget to breathe. When you've had enough return to Step 1 and come into Child's Pose for a rest.

Riding the Camel

The Camel ○ *Ustrasana*

The Camel posture is a magnificent backbend. With your dog sitting on your chest, you will be 'forced' to lift up through your breast bone, allowing the breath to open in a way that may feel unnatural and strenuous at first but, after a period of time and practice, you will feel like a weight has been taken off your chest as the diaphragm works to its full capacity. Backbends expand the breath and chest, invigorating the mind. They also stretch the spine, hips and shoulders. For your dog, this is another opportunity to connect with your breathing and gain trust in you.

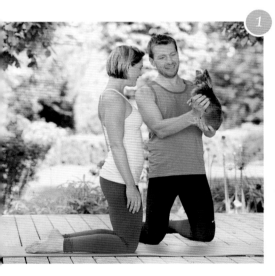

1   Kneel on the floor with your knees hip-distance apart. Keep your hips stacked over the knees, rotating the inner thighs inwards. Press your shins and the tops of your feet into the floor. Allow your Doga buddy to hold your dog until you are ready.

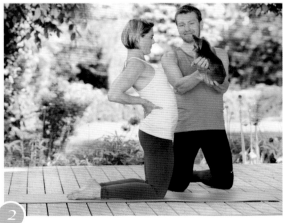

Exhale and rest your hands on your back with the palms just above your buttocks, fingers pointing down. Now ask your Doga buddy to place your dog on your chest. 2

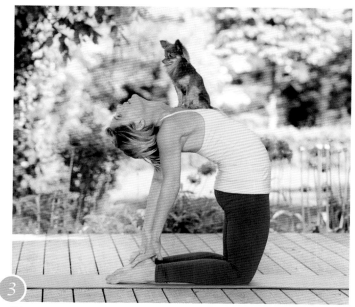

3

Maintain a high arch in your mid-spine. Exhale, reach your right hand to your right heel and then your left hand to your left heel. Inhale, lift the chest higher and roll your shoulders back and down. Relax your head back. Lift your breastbone and push the pelvis forwards, keeping the thighs vertical. Stay in this posture for as long as is comfortable, keeping your breathing smooth and even.

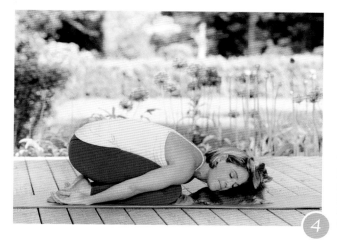

4

To exit, bring your hands onto the hips, inhale and lift your head back up, and allow your Doga buddy to take your dog off your chest. Exhale, sit back on your heels and breathe deeply. Rest in Child's Pose.

The Wagging Wheel

The Wheel ◯ *Urdva Dhanurasana*

The Wheel is all about trust and fun. The pose requires strength and flexibility from you, but calmness and trust from your dog, so it's best to save this until towards the end of a session when he's less excited. It's an impressive display of both your yogic and dogic skills.

This position is a real shoulder opener and also nurtures and awakens the spine. For you it's an invigorating pose, and for the dog it's a calming position. Having your dog there engages your abdomen wall, stabilizing your pelvis and reminding you of your core. He'll also help strengthen your legs in this position.

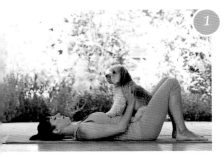

1. When your dog is calm, place him on your hips with his front paws on your chest. Hold him until you feel him relax, then lie back with your knees bent and your feet parallel, hips' width apart.

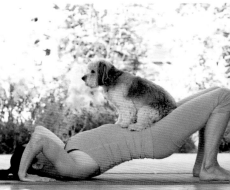

2. When you feel confident that he's happy in the position, let go of your dog and place your hands on the floor beside your ears, with fingertips pointing towards your shoulders. Pause for a moment so that you can be sure he's settled without your support.

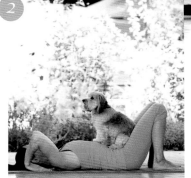

3. Inhale and press through your hands and feet, extending your tailbone forwards and lifting your hips towards the ceiling. The more slowly you can do this, the better, as your dog will feel unsteady. During your first few attempts, your dog is likely to jump off – if this happens, carry on with the pose and get a Doga buddy to place your dog on you (See box, opposite page).

helping hand

It's worth asking a Doga buddy to place your dog on your chest the first time you try this pose, so that both he and you can get used to the experience. Unless you are perfectly smooth when moving up into The Wheel, it's unlikely your dog will remain in place, but the more you practise with him, the more likely you'll both be happy in your roles.

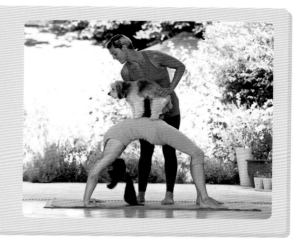

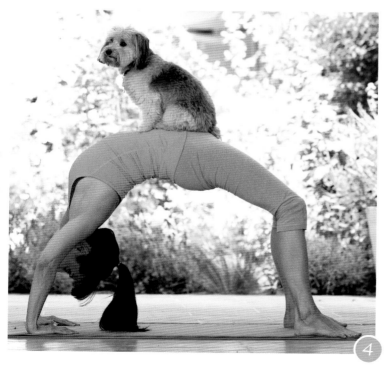

Continue to inhale as you straighten your arms and legs fully. Keep the weight evenly distributed through all four limbs. Gaze straight back and relax your neck. Hold the pose and breathe for several deep breaths.

4

May the Force Be With You

Advanced backbend sequence

This sequence is demanding: not only are you balancing your dog on your back, but it requires core strength and flexibility through the shoulders and hips. Backbends such as the Wheel are physically challenging but mentally rewarding. Only attempt this sequence once you are strong in your yoga practice. Be careful and mindful, and practise it after you have completed your regular warm-up of Sun Salutations (See pages 28–33) and some standing and forward bends.

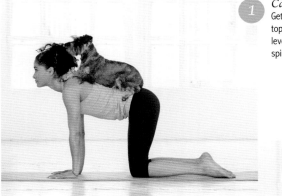

1 *Cat Stretch (Marjaryasana)*
Get your Doga buddy to place your dog on top of your mid spine. Keep your spine as level as a table top. Exhale and round your spine upwards.

Inhale and extend your spine towards the back of the room until your spine is straight again. **2**

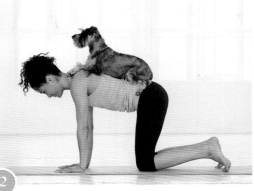

3 Downward Facing Dog (Adho Mukha Svanasana)

Inhale, engage your core and lift your sitting bones up towards the ceiling. Ensure your Doga buddy is there to steady your dog. Stay in Downward Facing Dog for 3–5 breaths, keeping your abdomen, arms and legs strong and engaged.

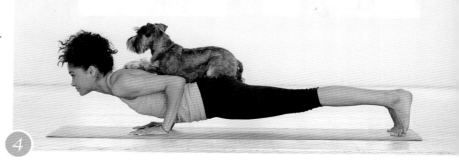

Four-limbed Staff Pose (Chaturranga Dandasana)

Fully and sharply exhale as you lower yourself down into Four-limbed Staff Pose. Hold the pose for a couple of breaths. 4

In Doga, the Bow
pose becomes the
Shopping Basket

5

Exhale and lower your navel
to the mat, pointing your toes
back. Lie on your stomach with
your arms alongside the torso
and your palms facing up.

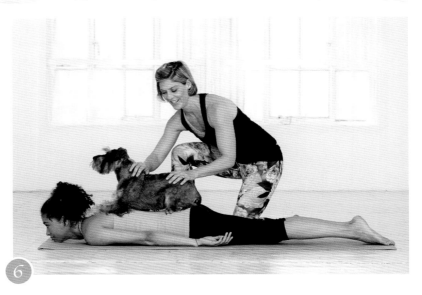

Ask your Doga buddy to
steady your dog. On an
exhale, bend the knees,
then reach back and take
hold of your ankles with
your hands. Keep the knees
hip-width apart. 6

The Bow (Dhanurasana)

Inhale, lift your chest and engage your core as you lift into the Bow. As you continue lifting the heels and thighs higher, draw your shoulder blades together to open the chest. Lift from your chest but try not to strain the neck and face. Use your abdomen muscles and inner thighs to support this deep extension in your spine. Breathe deeply and consistently for 3–5 breaths. Exhale, come down and rest for a few breaths.

8 Child's Pose (Balasana)

Push yourself up and back into Child's Pose and rest for a few breaths to stretch out your lower back muscles.

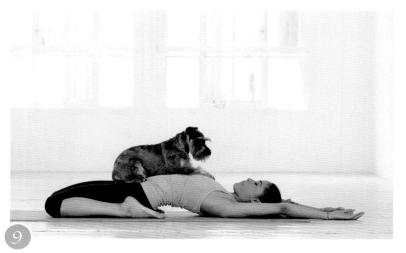

Reclining Hero (Supta Virasana)

Inhale and come back up. Place your dog on your upper thighs. Exhale and lower your hands to the floor. Continue to exhale as you descend backwards slowly, allowing your dog to rest on your navel, with his front paws on your chest. Your dog needs to sit comfortably. Ask your Doga buddy for help if necessary. Stay in Reclining Hero for 5–10 breaths to allow your hips and the backs of your legs to open. 9

The Wheel (Urdva Dhanurasana)

Now unfold your legs. You may have to cheat a little to wriggle yourself out of the pose, or, alternatively, take your dog off your chest and slowly come back up again. Now lie flat down on your back, bend your knees, keeping them hip-distance apart, and ensure your heels are in line with the buttock bones. Allow your dog to rest on your chest. Exhale and place your hands on the floor next to your ears. Keep your navel strong and engaged, using assistance from your Doga buddy. Inhale, lift up into Wheel and stay for 5–8 breaths.

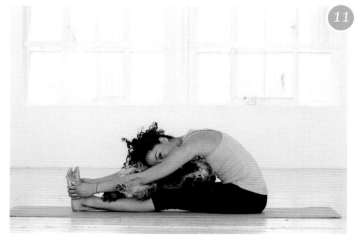

Seated Forward Bend (Paschimottanasana)

To come out of Wheel, engage your core and keep your legs strong as you bend the elbows and tuck in the chin as you lower yourself back down. Ensure the head is the last thing to release to the ground. If your dog jumps off during the process, let him. Come up into a seated position. Exhale, bend forwards from your torso and rest over your dog in a deep Forward Bend. Stay in this position as long as you need to and continue to breath deeply from your abdomen so your dog can engage with your breath.

Supine poses are excellent after backbends, as they bring your spine back to neutral. Lying on your back, you get a chance to ground yourself. The mind quietens and prepares for a meditative state. Lying back with your dog close to your chest is the ultimate 'bonding moment'.

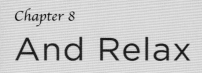

Chapter 8

And Relax

The Great Rejuvenators

Knees to Chest Pose ○ *Legs up the Wall Pose*

Knees to Chest Pose balances digestion and bowel movements and releases tension in the lower back. For your dog, this is a great opportunity to receive a hug and a massage, which helps with bonding. Legs up the Wall pose is one of the most powerful restorative poses, and is excellent before going to bed or if you had a stressful day. If you have no time for any other poses, do this one!

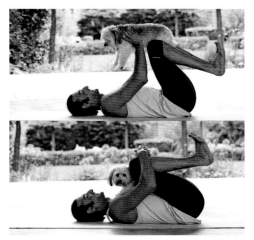

Legs up the Wall Pose (Viparita Karani)

Sit sideways with your right side against the wall. Place your dog on your lap. With one smooth movement, swing your legs up onto the wall and your shoulders and head lightly down to the floor. Close your eyes and allow the breath to soften and expand. Feel your legs drain and your mind empty, and enjoy the warmth and weight of your dog on your chest. Stay in this pose for 10–20 minutes, or as long as you feel necessary, then lower the heels and bring your knees towards the chest. Gently roll over onto your side and rest there for a while before coming up into seated posture.

Knees to Chest Pose (Apanasana)

Lie down on your back. Bring your knees to your chest and lift your dog up off the floor, with your hands under his armpits, and place him wherever he is most comfortable. If your dog is restless, just hold him on your knees and shins and bring them in.

Variation

If your dog is lying flat on your tummy, wrap your arms around your knees and interlace your fingers. Relax your neck and shoulders, feeling the weight of your knees drawing towards your chest. Avoid pulling your knees — let the weight of your dog do the work for you. Breathe deeply for 1–2 minutes, then roll over onto your side.

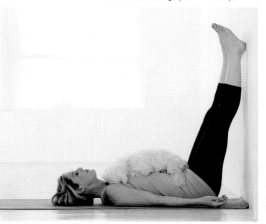

A Bridge with a View

Seated Bridge ○ *Setu Bandha Sarvangasana*

This posture strengthens the back of your body and stretches the back of your neck, making it an effective inversion as well as a backbend that prepares you for the Wheel. With your dog on your hips, you will have to engage the correct muscles in order to come into this full extension. With practice, you will find the ultimate moment of trust, when you can release your hands to the floor.

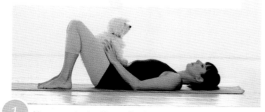

1 Lie on your back with your feet hip-distance apart and your knees bent at a right angle. Place your dog on your thighs and slide your hands under his armpits to provide support.

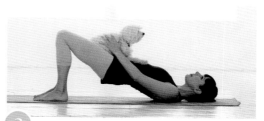

2 Exhale, press into the feet firmly and draw your shoulder blades together. Inhale and pick your pelvis off the ground while continuing to extend your tailbone forwards. Keep your knees stacked over your ankle bones.

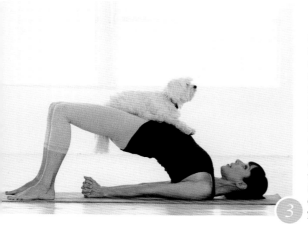

Continue to inhale and extend your tailbone until your hips are as high as they can go. Avoid straining your neck as you come up onto your shoulder blades. If you think your dog is comfortable and safe, release your hands and fold your arms behind your back, interlacing the fingers. Continue to press down through your forearms, keeping the hips pinned to the ceiling. Stay in this pose for 3–5 breaths. Make eye contact with your dog and breathe deeply using your abdomen, so your dog can feel you expanding, releasing and contracting. Exhale, then come down gently and release the pose until your back is flat on the ground. Draw your knees towards your chest and relax. Follow up Seated Bridge with Knees to Chest Pose (see opposite page), which provides a great counterpose for 3 your lower back.

Happy Puppy Pose

Happy Baby Pose ○ *Ananda Balasana*

A deep hip opener that helps alleviate stress and fatigue, this is a classic restorative pose. Like an infant being pampered, we can feel a sense of joy and easy in Happy Baby Pose. The weight of your dog against your chest or navel will coax your mind to explore the breath and the body in greater depth. This pose should enable both of you to find comfort and trust in each other.

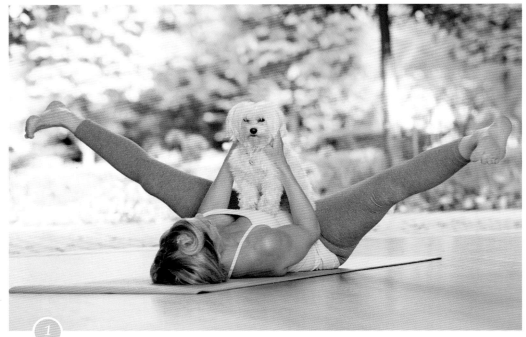

1 Lie on your back with your legs raised up and held wide apart. Place your dog on your navel, preferably flat on his belly, or else sitting on all fours.

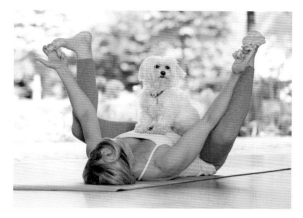

Variation
Keep your knees bent if you
can't straighten your legs all the
way in this position.

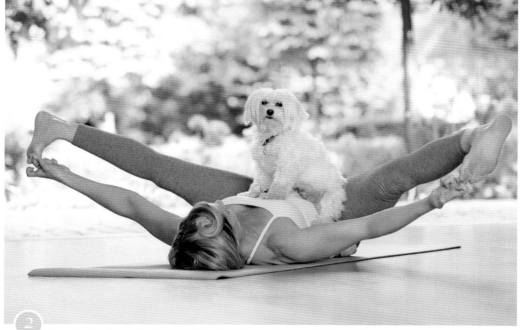

On an inhalation flex your heels and grab hold of your big toes. Coax the thighs in towards the torso and down towards the floor as you lengthen the spine, releasing the tailbone towards the floor. Hold the pose steadily for 30–60 seconds, then release the feet back to the floor with an exhale and rest for a few breaths.

Riding on a Fish Tail

Fish Pose ○ *Matsyasana*

This pose is frequently used as a counterpose to Legs up the Wall pose because it reverses the position of the cervial spine from extreme flexion to extreme extension. This backbend releases shoulder and neck tension and opens and expands the chest. Your Dogi can enjoy a ride on your fishtail as he connects with the waves of your breath – imagine swimming together in the deep blue sea, alongside mermaids and dolphins.

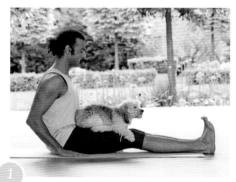

1. Sitting upright, with legs extended, and settle your dog on the tops of your thighs, either facing away from you or towards you, whichever way he is comfortable. Keep your inner thighs rolled in and your toes pointing up.

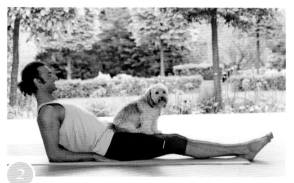

2. Exhale, come down onto your forearms, preferably sliding your hands under your buttocks, squeezing your elbows together. Roll the inner thighs closer together and point your toes. Gaze at your dog.

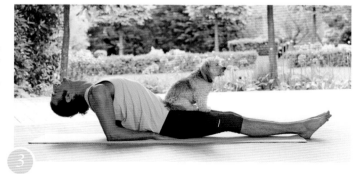

3. Inhale and lift the sternum, then exhale and take your head back. Gaze between your eyebrows. Keep breathing deeply for 3–5 breaths. To release the pose, inhale, lift your head and gently push yourself back to a seated position.

Doga Snooze Pose

Corpse Pose ○ *Savasana*

The perfect pose with which to end your Doga session, the Corpse Pose helps restore the central nervous system. In this posture you experience gravity pulling you down to the earth – let everything go and quieten the mind. Stay in this pose for at least 5 minutes. Then roll over onto your right side and rest for a few breaths before coming back up to a seated positition.

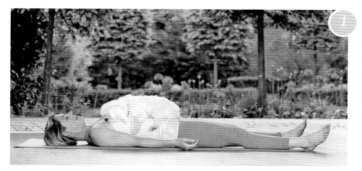

Lie flat on your back, with your feet hip-width apart, palms facing upwards. Allow your dog to rest on your belly. Let your fingers and toes uncurl. Visualize a straight line from the crown of your head all the way through your spine and down into your tailbone. Imagine you had a 'doggie tail': with each exhalation, lengthen your tail towards the front of the room. Relax your forehead, the root of your tongue, the back of the eyes and the inner ears.

modification

This variation of the Corpse Pose is suitable for those with lower back problems. Lie flat on your back, your arms out to the side, and bring your heels towards the buttocks, keeping your knees at a 45-degree angle and your toes turned slightly inwards. Allow your dog to rest on your belly. Imagine that you can breathe in calm, then exhale and breathe out stress. This way both you and your dog experience total peace, as your dog rides the waves of your breath.

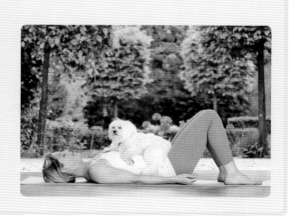

Massage

Massaging your dog can have numerous benefits for both Dogi and Yogi. For the Yogi, petting your dog releases the hormone oxytocin, which triggers feelings of happiness and relief from stress and depression. And, for the Dogi, receiving a massage can be an excellent way of reducing pain and anxiety. Most importantly, massaging your dog enhances your natural bond and creates trust between you. The benefits of massage include:

○ Increases circulation and flexibility
○ The release of feel-good endorphins
○ It develops and maintains muscles tone
○ It can reduce stiffness and joint discomfort
○ Improved sleep and digestion
○ It combats anxiety, hyperactivity and restlessness.

The following massage exercises, except for Flexion and Extension of Paw Massage on page 135, can be used at any point during your Doga practice, especially in restorative and counterposes.

Top to Tail Massage

Start your massage practice by repeatedly stroking your dog, all the way from the top of his head to his tail, gently but thoroughly. You will both find this experience very relaxing.

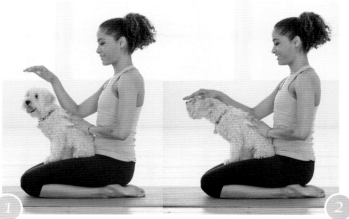

Sit back on your heels. Keep your spine straight. Place your dog on your knees, facing away from you. Make sure he's sitting comfortably on his front paws. If your dog is larger, sit in Wide-legged Seated Pose and place him between your legs, facing away from you.

Begin by lightly resting your hand, palm flat, on top of your dog's head. Make slow, sweeping movements down his spine to the tail. Repeat several times, alternating hands each time. You can gradually increase your pressure if your dog is comfortable with this, but avoid pressing straight down on the lower part of his back. Finish by resting one hand at the base of your dog's head and the other hand on your dog's hips.

Joint Massage

Make sure not to use too much pressure through the fingers when massaging the tender muscles around your dog's joints, whether it is around the front legs or hip bones, as dogs experience a lot of soreness and stiffness in their muscle joints. Using only the soft pads of your fingertips, and apply very light pressure through your middle and index fingers when massaging these areas. Keep your third and index fingers close together and make long, sweeping motions in the direction in which your dog's fur grows.

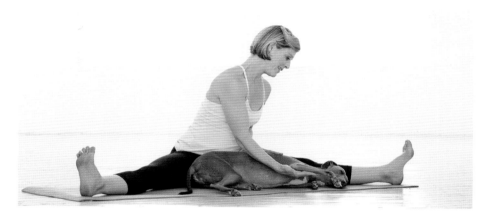

Front Legs

Slide your hand under your dog's leg, with palm facing upwards, to support the joint. Starting from the top of the leg bone, brush the index and third fingers of your other hand over the muscles alongside the shoulder joint. Avoid touching the bone. When you've finished with the upper leg, apply the same technique to the foreleg. Finish by picking up your dog's paw and squeezing gently. Repeat on the other side,

Back legs

Work your fingers the same way as for the front legs along the muscles that surround the hip joint. If your dog is too sensitive in the hip area, try doing these motions without any pressure. If that's still too uncomfortable for your pet, try doing the motion just above the hips and legs. Even though you may not be touching your animal, you will still benefit from the energetic exchange and intention.

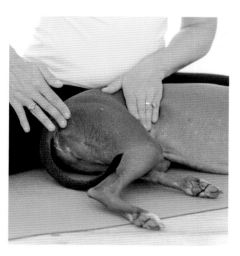

Neck massage

Most dogs hold a large amount of muscular tension behind and under their ears, so a careful, gentle neck massage can make him feel good. You can apply more pressure if you see that your dog is enjoying the experience.

Sit crossed-legged or in Wide-legged Seated Pose. Place your dog in front of you. Place the thumb and index finger of both hands inside the nape of your dog's neck, just where the base of his head and neck connect. Apply pressure through your fingers and massage the muscles around the neck joint in small, circular motions. You can work your way up the length of his neck to the base of the head. Go back down in the same circular motions. Continue for 3–5 minutes in total.

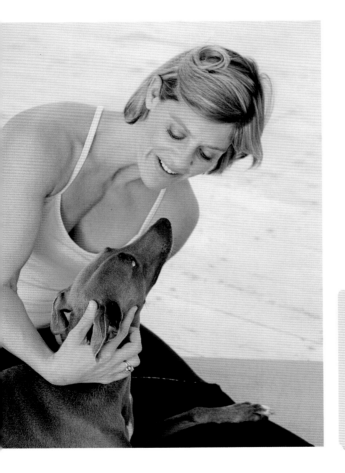

health note

If you feel a lot of heat around the joints, it could be a sign of muscular distress or joint issues and you should consult your vet.

Flexion and Extension of Paw

Working with your dog's natural range of movement in the leg and hip bone can prevent future disease like arthritis or stiffness in the joints.

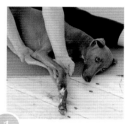

1 Sit in an upright position with your shoulders relaxed. Your dog should be lying on his side, facing away from you. Slide your right palm underneath his elbow joint. With your left hand, gently support the weight of his front paws, with your palm facing upwards.

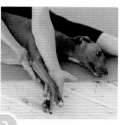

2 Keeping your right hand flat and fingers together, press your third and index finger into the bony elbow joint. Adding pressure into that joint will flex the front paw automatically. Keep soft pressure until the muscle extends fully. Hold for 30 seconds.

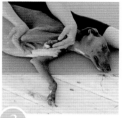

3 Hold your dog's paw and press it softly back towards his shoulder joint, with your right hand supporting his elbow. With a flat palm, apply more pressure and press the paw further back into his shoulder joint. Hold the flexion for 30 seconds.

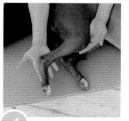

4 Repeat Steps 1–3 on the back leg. Place your right hand, palm upwards, underneath your dog's ankle joint and your left hand underneath his knee joint for support. Make sure that his muscles are relaxed before you move on to the next step.

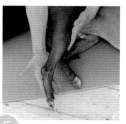

5 With your left palm, gently press into his knee cap, while your right hand supports the weight of his back paw. Progressively add gentle pressure until the muscles of his back leg automatically extend out. Hold the extension for 20–30 seconds.

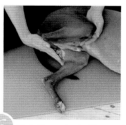

6 Tuck his paw back with your right hand and continue to press into the hip joint. Hold for 20–30 seconds. Then repeat the whole sequence on his other side.

Howling

Howling is one of your dog's basic instincts, inherited from his wolf ancestors, who howled to make their presence known and to tell the pack there was hunting to do. Like wolves, dogs try to imitate each other's pitch and to amplify the sound to create the illusion that there are more pack members.

It's common for dogs to howl at the sound of a police car's siren, a fire engine, occasionally even the television. If dogs hear something that sounds like a howl to them, they will instinctively start to howl. Howling can also be a sign of happiness: the dog is communicating his joy to you and the rest of his pack.

Creating Beneficial Sounds

Dogs have super-sensitive hearing. When a dog hears a sudden sound, he stops what he's doing and locates the source of the sound. A wailing siren or exploding firework can trigger the fight-or-flight in-stinct – in some cases, these noises make dogs go 'barking mad'.

However, you can create sounds that are beneficial to your dog. *Bijas*, or 'mystical seeds', are one-note syllables that affect the central *nadi* or channel of the nervous system – both yours and that of your dog. Similar to lullabies that a mother sings to her child, you can sing *bijas* to your dog to calm him down and make him less anxious and agitated. It is advisable to use deep breathing when creating the sound, so that it comes from the navel/abdomen rather than the head region, as a high-pitched noise may hurt your dog's ears.

Aum

The best-known single-syllable *bija* in the Hindu tradition is the sacred sound of Aum, or Om. According to the ancient Vedas, Aum is the sound that vibrates through and permeates the universe. Chanting this sound brings peace and calm to the body, mind and soul by merging the vibrations of the body with those of the universe.

Most of the mantras in yoga that derives from Hinduism start with the word Aum, which in itself is a complete mantra or 'sound seed', with a strong vibration that can influence all living beings. Patanjali, the father of modern yoga, wrote in his Sutras that, if a person focused his or her mind on chanting Aum and contemplating its meaning, he or she, too, could achieve enlightenment.

How to chant 'Aum'

Sit cross-legged or in Lotus pose on a cushion or a folded blanket, with a straight spine and your hands on your knees, with palms facing upwards. Place your dog on your lap or let him lie next to you, if he prefers. Ensure that he's in a peaceful, calm and relaxed state before beginning the exercise. If he wanders off during this exercise, let him be.

1 Take a deep inhalation through the nose and, on the exhalation, chant 'Aaa...', making the sound from the depths of your belly. Feel the vibrations of the sound in your abdomen. After you have fully exhaled, relax for a few seconds.

2 Inhale and, while exhaling, chant 'Ooo...'. Feel the vibrations in your chest and neck. It doesn't matter if your pitch is slightly different than before, as long as it's not so high that it distresses your dog. After you have fully exhaled, relax for a few seconds.

3 Inhale again, a long, slow breath. While exhaling, chant 'Mmm....'. Feel the vibrations in your head and neck. Exhale and relax for a few seconds.

4 Now inhale again and, while exhaling, chant 'Aummmmm'. About 80 percent of the exhalation should be for 'Au' and the other twenty percent for 'mmm'.

Repeat the sound 5–10 times. You can increase the number over time. When you have finished, close your eyes and draw your mind inwards. See how you and your dog feel. Take 5–10 deep breaths, then open your eyes. Check your dog's response to the vibrations of the sound: is he enjoying it? If he pricks up his ears and begins to wince, you may want to decrease the volume and turn it into a whisper. Remember that your dog needs time to familiarize himself with this sound.

Once your dog is used to the sound of you chanting 'Aum', you can add the peace mantra Om Shanti (see below) to your yoga practice.

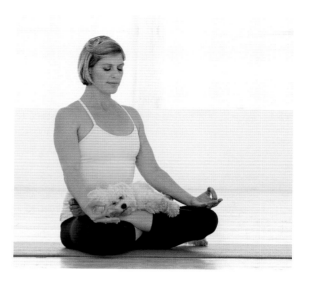

Chanting Om Shanti

Om śāntih śāntih śāntih is a Sanskrit mantra that is used after prayers, meditation or yoga. It comes from the word *sham*, meaning 'to be at peace', so Shanti means calm, tranquillity, peace, permanent satisfaction, fulfillment, contentment or stillness. Shanti is repeated three times to bring peace to the three realms of existence: the Phyiscal (*Adhi-Bhautika*), the Divine (*Adhi-Daivika*) and the Internal (*Adhyaatmika*).

Take a deep inhalation, then on the exhalation, try to recite the *Om śāntih śāntih śāntih* mantra on one breath. Take a few breaths, then recite it again. The more we practise, the better we become.

Feel free to add these mantras at the beginning of your practice, to settle yourself and your dog, or use them to complete your Doga practice.

Index

Relaxing feet

For Sam and Peggy, and all dogs that are hoping for a new home.

An Hachette UK Company
www.hachette.co.uk

First published in Great Britain in 2015
by Hamlyn, a division of Octopus Publishing
Group Ltd
Carmelite House
50 Victoria Embankment
London EC4Y 0DZ
www.octopusbooks.co.uk
www.octopusbooksusa.com

Distributed in the US by
Hachette Book Group
1290 Avenue of the Americas
4th and 5th Floors
New York, NY 10020

Distributed in Canada by
Canadian Manda Group
664 Annette St.
Toronto, Ontario, Canada M6S 2C8

ISBN 978-0-60062-892-7
A CIP catalogue record for this book is available
from the British Library

Printed and bound in China
10 9 8 7 6 5 4 3 2 1

Editorial Director Trevor Davies
Project Editor Alex Stetter
Deputy Art Director Yasia Leedham-Williams
Designer Isabel de Cordova
Photographer Ruth Jenkinson
Hair and Make-up Artists Victoria Barnes, Roisin
Donaghy
Production Controller Meskerem Berhane

Author's Acknowledgements

Special thanks to my parents, Frances and Mehdi
Djahanguiri, for their love, support, sound advice,
madness and creativity that helped me visualize
and dream 'the dream'. I love you. To my beautiful
brother Thierry... this is for you. To Uncle John and
Auntie Jean, for allowing me to jam their photo-
copy machine.

A very big thank you to Michelle Spurr and Mina
and of course the first doginis, Holly and Poppy.
To my dearest friend, Marc Baker, who spotted the
potential of Doga, to Harish Patel, for his friendship,
enthusiasm and professional advice, and to Ira from
All Dogs Matter, for giving me my first Doga gig.
Futhermore I'd like to thank Claudia Polly Bream,
Rick Alancroft and Penelope Dudley, Richard Hillier
and Sharron Hines for their ongoing support.

Thank you to my 'Cover Girl' and friend Jay Read
for her help with the editing, and to all the other
models in ths book: Shiraz Haq, Genevieve
Capovilla, Mark Sroczynski and Lily Baruah.
Thank you to Dima Yeremenko and his dogs, and
to Angel, Lucky and Baxter.

To my wonderful editor Trevor Davies, for offering
me the chance to write this book and making the
journey so easy and enjoyable, to Alex Stetter for
her editing skills and to my agent Sophie at MBA.
A special thank you to Ruth Jenkinson, the coolest
photographer in town and her creative team.

Thank you to those who supported the idea of
Doga: the Pet Spa at Harrods, Vicki Marie Cossar,
Joanne Good, Anna Webb, Cheska Hull and many,
many more. To my Yoga teachers Anna Wise and
Hamish Hendry and everyone at AYL, and to Katie
Mutton from Yoga Team for her advice. I'd like to
thank all my clients and doggie friends who have
participated in Doga, with a special thank you to
Marianne and Lily, Petrina Cutchey and Brooke,
Alex and Benji, Yuko and Poppy, Flick Thorley and
Walley and Lulu and Sofia Gomez. Without you,
there would be no Doga.

And last but not least, thank you to my little family,
my canine companion Robbie and Samantha the
cat. You're both the apple of my eye.